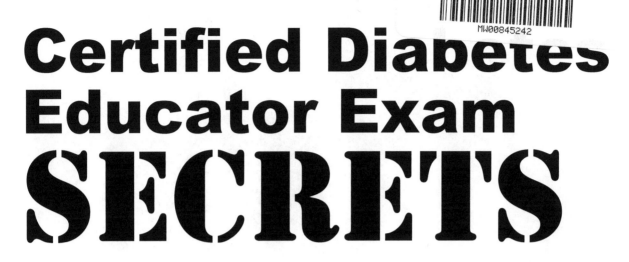

Certified Diabetes Educator Exam
SECRETS

Study Guide
Your Key to Exam Success

CDE Test Review for the
Certified Diabetes Educator Exam

Published by
Mometrix Test Preparation
CDE Exam Secrets Test Prep Team

Written and edited by the CDE Exam Secrets Test Prep Staff

Printed in the United States of America

This paper meets the requirements of ANSI/NISO Z39.48-1992 (Permanence of Paper).

Mometrix offers volume discount pricing to institutions. For more information or a price quote, please contact our sales department at sales@mometrix.com or 888-248-1219.

ISBN 13: 978-1-60971-301-0
ISBN 10:1-60971-301-X

Dear Future Exam Success Story:

Congratulations on your purchase of our study guide. Our goal in writing our study guide was to cover the content on the test, as well as provide insight into typical test taking mistakes and how to overcome them.

Standardized tests are a key component of being successful, which only increases the importance of doing well in the high-pressure high-stakes environment of test day. How well you do on this test will have a significant impact on your future, and we have the research and practical advice to help you execute on test day.

The product you're reading now is designed to exploit weaknesses in the test itself, and help you avoid the most common errors test takers frequently make.

How to use this study guide

We don't want to waste your time. Our study guide is fast-paced and fluff-free. We suggest going through it a number of times, as repetition is an important part of learning new information and concepts.

First, read through the study guide completely to get a feel for the content and organization. Read the general success strategies first, and then proceed to the content sections. Each tip has been carefully selected for its effectiveness.

Second, read through the study guide again, and take notes in the margins and highlight those sections where you may have a particular weakness.

Finally, bring the manual with you on test day and study it before the exam begins.

Your success is our success

We would be delighted to hear about your success. Send us an email and tell us your story. Thanks for your business and we wish you continued success.

Sincerely,

Mometrix Test Preparation Team

Need more help? Check out our flashcards at:
http://MometrixFlashcards.com/CertifiedDiabetesEducator

TABLE OF CONTENTS

Top 20 Test Taking Tips

1. Carefully follow all the test registration procedures
2. Know the test directions, duration, topics, question types, how many questions
3. Setup a flexible study schedule at least 3-4 weeks before test day
4. Study during the time of day you are most alert, relaxed, and stress free
5. Maximize your learning style; visual learner use visual study aids, auditory learner use auditory study aids
6. Focus on your weakest knowledge base
7. Find a study partner to review with and help clarify questions
8. Practice, practice, practice
9. Get a good night's sleep; don't try to cram the night before the test
10. Eat a well balanced meal
11. Know the exact physical location of the testing site; drive the route to the site prior to test day
12. Bring a set of ear plugs; the testing center could be noisy
13. Wear comfortable, loose fitting, layered clothing to the testing center; prepare for it to be either cold or hot during the test
14. Bring at least 2 current forms of ID to the testing center
15. Arrive to the test early; be prepared to wait and be patient
16. Eliminate the obviously wrong answer choices, then guess the first remaining choice
17. Pace yourself; don't rush, but keep working and move on if you get stuck
18. Maintain a positive attitude even if the test is going poorly
19. Keep your first answer unless you are positive it is wrong
20. Check your work, don't make a careless mistake

Assessment

Learning / Self Care Behaviors

Learning Needs Assessment

Prior to teaching, assess the following areas:
- Previous learning, current level of knowledge and health beliefs about diabetes – "Tell me what you already know about diabetes."
- Patient's goals – "What would you like to learn?"; "What goals do you have for various health measures such as blood pressure, blood sugar, lipid values and bodyweight)?"
- Attitudes and feelings about diabetes and the educational program – "How important is education to you?" "How can education help you?"
- Preferred learning styles – "How do you prefer to learn (e.g., video, reading, listening, hands-on, etc)?" "Do you have any conditions that could affect how you learn (e.g., hearing loss, vision loss, low reading level, second language)?"
- Psychological status – "How are you feeling mentally?" Assess for depression, anxiety, stress or other factors that could get in the way of learning.
- Social and cultural factors – "Who else should learn with you?"
- Readiness and willingness – "On a scale from 1 – 10, how ready are you to learn (0 = not at all ready; 10 = as ready as I could possibly be)?"

Characteristics of the Adult Learner

The adult learner:

- Is self-directed. The adult prefers to have a say in the learning agenda. It is helpful to start by asking the client what he or she would like to learn.
- Needs a reason to learn. The adult wants information that is useful. Teaching content should focus on specific problems rather than comprehensive subject matter.
- Prefers information that is personalized and relevant. Curriculums for adult education should incorporate past experiences of participants. Time should be spent on discussing problems that the participant has identified.
- Is an active learner. Programs should include plenty of opportunity for sharing and problem-solving.

Adult Diabetes Self-Management Education

Group discussions allow learners to be active participants in their learning. These also make the program more relevant by allowing group members to select content that is important to them. Group scission provides a forum for practicing problem-solving skills. Group leaders need to be able to keep the group focused and prevent one or two members from dominating.

Demonstration is a preferred strategy for tactile learners. Skills such as blood sugar testing and injecting insulin can be learned by demonstration. The participant should provide a return demonstration to asses learning and receive feedback.

Audiovisual aids help to hold interest by engaging multiple senses and learning styles. Examples include food models, PowerPoint presentations, flip charts, videos and slides. Certain audiovisual aids can be especially useful for clients with low literacy.

Role playing engages learners and allows them to be active in the learning process. Role plays are helpful in practicing problem-solving skills.

<u>Goals and Content of Diabetes Self-Management Education</u>
The American Diabetes Association and the American Association of Diabetes Educators have set evidence-based standards for the content and outcome of diabetes self-management education (DSME).

The goals and objectives of DSME include enabling people with diabetes to make informed decisions and actively participate as much as possible in their own care. These objectives are met by programs that provide training in self-care behavior, problem-solving and collaboration with healthcare providers.

Content of DSME programs include:
- Diabetes disease process
- Food and nutrition
- Physical activity and exercise
- Medication
- Self-monitoring of blood glucose
- Acute complications, including prevention and treatment
- Chronic complications, including prevention and treatment
- Psychological and social adjustment to diabetes
- Problem-solving
- Setting goals
- Pregnancy planning and preconception care, if applicable

Health Belief Model

Components of the Health Belief Model include:

- Perceived benefits. People who feel that they will reap benefits from engaging in self-care behaviors will be more likely to learn and apply these skills.
- Perceived costs. Costs include financial expense, time spent and energy invested. People who perceive that the benefits outweigh the costs are more likely to engage in the learning process and make the necessary changes.
- Severity of diabetes and complications. Disability, illness and loss of productivity are markers of disease severity. People who believe that diabetes is a serious condition are more likely to accept education.
- Susceptibility. Those who perceive that the negative consequences of diabetes can happen to them are more willing to engage in education. Those who feel they have "borderline" or "mild" diabetes may not believe that education is necessary for them.

According to research, perceived susceptibility and disease severity are the strongest predictors for behavior change.

Locus of Control

Locus of control refers to one's belief about who or what controls health outcomes. The Locus of Control Theory provides three possible orientations for this belief system:

Internal locus of control
- The person believes that he or she holds most of the power in determining the outcome of a health event. A person with diabetes who has an internal locus of control will feel that his or her actions make a difference.

External locus of control
- Also known as "powerful other" orientation.
- The person believes that others have the most power in determining their outcome. Healthcare providers are often perceived as powerful others. Those having this orientation would believe that their doctor plays the most important role in their health care. Other significant people in the person's life can be perceived as the powerful other.

Chance orientation
- The person believes that fate, luck or chance determine his or her outcome.

Assessing locus of control can help identify those who do not recognize the important role that self-management plays in positive diabetes outcomes.

Comparison of Theories

<u>Health Belief Model, Locus of Control Theory and Self-Efficacy Theory</u>
Health Belief Model – People are more likely to engage in health behaviors if they perceive that the benefits of taking action outweigh the costs. In addition, this model suggests that people are more likely to adhere to self-care practices if they believe that their condition is serious enough to warrant behavior change and that they are susceptible to poor outcomes if they do not practice these behaviors.

Locus of Control Theory – People with an internal locus of control are more likely to make health behavior change than those with an external locus of control. People with an internal locus of control believe that their health outcome is dependent upon their own actions rather than the actions of others or chance.

Self-Efficacy Theory – People who feel confident that they can perform health behaviors are more likely to engage in these behaviors than people who lack this confidence.

Each of these models helps educators assess the belief systems that determine adoption of health behaviors and adherence to diabetes self-care practices.

Learning Style Preferences

Most people have one or two predominant learning styles. Assessing a person's preferred learning style can help in tailoring a program to the individual's needs.

- Visual learners prefer to see the material being presented. Programs should make use of graphics, charts, models, pictures, books, videos and demonstrations.
- Auditory learners prefer to hear the material being presented. Programs for auditory learners include audio tapes and discussions.
- Tactile learners like a hands-on approach. Demonstrations return demonstrations and other show-and-tell methods will appeal to this learner.
- Social learners learn best in a group environment. These learners will benefit from group classes and workshops where interaction and sharing occur. Referral to community resources can also be beneficial.
- Solitary learners prefer to learn 1:1 or independently. Providing reading material and web-based resources are best for these learners.
- Low literacy clients present challenges as traditional education normally involves reading material. Programs can be adapted for people with low literacy by using pictorial handouts, video tapes and demonstrations. Individual teaching sessions may be necessary for the person with low literacy.

Low Literacy

Assessment can be difficult as many people with low literacy are ashamed. Building trust is key. Approach the client in a way that normalizes the situation. For example, begin by saying "I have had a lot of clients who had trouble reading the handouts they were given. How are you doing with those?"

Ask clients what are the best learning methods for them. Do they prefer videos, 1:1 discussion and handouts with lots of pictures?

Start with modest goals for learning, focusing on the most important and basic information first. Work up to material that is more complex.

Personalize the content, using phrases such as "your meal plan" and "your diabetes."

Use repetition freely and periodically ask the client to recall what has been discussed.

Use visual aids, mnemonic devices and analogies to help the client mentally organize the material.

Culturally Competent Diabetes Education

Cultural sensitivity involves understanding and accepting that others may have differing views of health care than the educator. Education that is culturally sensitive is more relevant to the client and promotes a more trusting relationship with the educator.

A thorough assessment includes gathering information about how clients view diabetes and their care from a cultural standpoint.

Cultural perspectives to be included in the assessment:
- Food preferences, including everyday foods, celebratory foods and foods used for religious purposes
- Role of fasting, if applicable
- Perceived cause of diabetes
- Perceived reason for why diabetes developed
- Perceived significance of diabetes
- Fears related to having diabetes

The educator cannot be expected to be an expert on every culture but instead to be sensitive that differences exist. The educator can be honest with clients in sharing that he or she would like to learn more about their cultures.

Depression in Diabetes Self-Management

Studies show that depression negatively affects self-care practice and outcomes.

Rates of depression among people with diabetes are high. Approximately 1 in 5 people with diabetes suffer from depression, although it is often not diagnosed.

Diabetes educators can screen for depression by asking a series of questions. If the client has 5 or more symptoms for a period of 2 weeks or more, he or she should be further evaluated for treatment of depression.

Screening questions for depression include:
- Do you feel sad much of the day, on most days?
- Have you gained or lost weight without trying?
- Do you have trouble falling asleep or do you sleep too much?
- Do you feel anxious most days?
- Are you low on energy most days?
- Have you lost interest or pleasure in things that you usually like?
- Do you feel guilty or worthless?
- Are you having trouble concentrating or making decisions?
- Do you think about death and dying a lot?
- Have you thought about suicide or made any such plans?

Economic Factors in Diabetes Self-Care

People with diabetes pay about three times more for out-of-pocket medical expenditures than those without diabetes.

Poverty can affect the person's ability to have the food, shelter and other resources necessary for proper self-management.

A comprehensive assessment includes asking the patient directly if he or she has the resources needed to practice diabetes self-care.

Community resources may include:
- Government medical programs such as Medicare and Medicaid
- Government food programs such as food stamps and WIC
- Local groups, such as the Lions Club, that may help those with visual impairment
- Low-cost or free diabetes education programs in the community
- Community food banks
- State vocational training resources

Family and Social Support in Diabetes Self-Care

Diabetes self-care pervades all aspects of the person's life and much of it takes place within a social context. Family and friends can have a significant impact on a person's self-care behavior.
- The major social influence on children is parents.
- The major social influence on adolescents is peers.
- The major social influences on adults are spouses, friends, co-workers and family members.

Social influences can enhance self-care if significant people are supportive. People are more likely to engage in positive self-care behavior when supported by their social network.

Social influence can have a negative impact if others are not supportive or undermine self-care efforts.

Social assessment includes finding out:
- Who helps with diabetes management
- Who hinders diabetes management
- What is needed for feeling supported
- Where additional support could be found
- How the healthcare provider can help increase social support resources

Diabetic with Physical Limitations

Many people who have had a stroke will need to learn how to do many self-care tasks one-handed. Occupational therapists are trained to help people perform activities of daily living as independently as possible.

Adaptive devices are available for testing blood sugar and for drawing and injecting insulin.

Social and family support is important, as significant others may be needed to pre-draw insulin syringes. The diabetes educator may be called upon to teach insulin preparation and care to families and caregivers of stroke victims.

Patients who have had amputations need support in dealing with limited mobility. Education on exercise as an integral part of diabetes management will need to be modified. Wheelchair bound clients can be encouraged to move as much as possible and to use light handheld weights or soup cans to exercise the upper body.

Visually Impaired

Assess ability to read printed information and medication labels.
- Effect of print size
- Effect of lighting
- Use of magnifying devices

Assess ability to read syringe markings.
- Effect of syringe size and size of syringe markings
- Effect of lighting
- Use of syringe magnifier
- Request demonstration of drawing insulin into syringe to correct amount AND/OR evaluate cost/benefit of using insulin pen, premixed insulin or prefilled syringes as needed.

Assess ability to self-monitor blood sugar.
- Request demonstration.
- Assess need and cost/benefit of using talking meter as needed.

Assess ability to verbalize correct timing, frequency and dose of prescribed insulin.

Assess ability to correctly inject insulin and request demonstration.

Assess understanding of causes, prevention, recognition and treatment of hypoglycemia and ability to respond to low blood sugar.

Physical Health Status

Physical health can affect a person's ability to engage in self-care behavior.

An acutely ill person may not be ready to learn and may be unable to concentrate on education.

Chronic illness can interfere with the ability to meet the challenges of diabetes self-care on a day-to-day basis. Complex medication regimens may need to be addressed and the potential for drug interactions considered.

People who are acutely or chronically ill may need shorter teaching sessions and recommendations may need to be modified or adapted. For example, the exercise recommendation may need to be modified or adapted for people who have neuropathy or hypertension.

Visual impairment can affect the ability to safely self-administer medications or insulin. Adaptive equipment, such as talking blood glucose meters and syringe magnifiers, are available for those with visual impairment.

Transtheoretical Model of Behavior Change

<u>Stages</u>
Pre-contemplation
- The person is not actively thinking about making any behavioral changes. This may be due to believing that the changes are not important or achievable or that the costs of change outweigh the benefits. If asked, the person would say that they are not planning to make any changes in the next 6 months.

Contemplation
- The person is thinking about making changes within the next 6 months, but has not made any changes yet.

Preparation
- The person has decided to change and is making plans to do so. For example, he or she has begun researching weight loss programs but has not yet started.

Action
- The person has started making the changes within the past 6 months.

Maintenance
- The person has made the changes and maintained them for 6 months or more.

The progression through these stages is not always linear and relapse is common. Recycling is a term used when a person goes back to a previous stage after relapse.

<u>Stage-Matched Interventions</u>

Pre-contemplation
- The person may actively resist change.
- Help client identify feelings and beliefs in a supportive way.

Contemplation
- The person may be ambivalent about change.
- Build confidence and support efforts.

Preparation
- Patient begins to visualize future self.
- Help with setting short and long-term goals.
- Provide encouragement and resources.

Action
- Patient is practicing new behaviors.
- Help strengthen client's commitment to the new behavior.
- Assist with problem-solving.

Maintenance
- The person has engaged in the new behavior for 6 or more months.
- Continue to support behaviors and self-efficacy.

Relapse
- The person has returned to any of the other earlier stages of change.
- Help client overcome feelings of failure.
- Avoid showing signs of disappointment or annoyance.
- Explore causes of relapse.
- Encourage movement to the next stage of change.

Self-Efficacy

Self-efficacy refers to a person's level of confidence in his or her ability to perform a behavior or set of behaviors.

Studies show that people with diabetes who have high self-efficacy tend to be more active in self-care, have better emotional health and maintain better glycemic control than those with low self-efficacy.

Assessing self-efficacy can help target areas of educational need.

The Diabetes Empowerment Scale (DES) is a 28-item questionnaire that measures diabetes self-efficacy.

Informal assessment of self-efficacy can include asking clients how confident they feel in performing specific diabetes-related behaviors such as checking blood sugar, eating the right amount of carbohydrate or responding to low blood sugar. Using a scale of 0 – 10 is recommended when asking the client to rate confidence (i.e. 0 = not all confident; 10 = very confident).

Newly Diagnosed Client with Diabetes

Initial diabetes education should begin as soon as feasible. This may be in the hospital or outpatient setting. Before beginning initial education, it is important to assess:

- Current health status
- Baseline understanding of the diabetes diagnosis and its implications
- Attitudes and beliefs about diabetes and self-care
- Emotional response to diagnosis and readiness to learn
- Current level of knowledge and skill related to diabetes self-care
- Age
- Functional status
- Preferred learning style
- Home/social situation and identification of helpers
- Cultural influences and language

Reassessment is recommended at later stages to evaluate adjustment and assimilation of self-care behavior.

Type 1 and Type 2 Diabetes Assessment

Type 1 diabetes – The patient often presents with abrupt onset of illness. Symptoms of hyperglycemia include polyuria, polydipsia, extreme hunger, weakness and recent history of unexplained weight loss. If ketoacidosis is present, symptoms may include dehydration, tachycardia, orthostatic hypotension and abdominal pain. The patient may also present with fruity acetone breath. Patients who present with type 1 diabetes are often younger than the age of 30 with a lean body type.

Type 2 diabetes. Typically, patients are over the age of 40 when diagnosed with type 2 diabetes, but onset in children and young adults is increasingly more common. The patient may exhibit no signs of hyperglycemia, as the diagnosis is often an incidental finding. Family history of diabetes, excess body weight and sedentary lifestyle are risk factors for type 2 diabetes. Certain ethnic groups have higher incidence of type 2 diabetes, namely American Indians, Alaska Natives, Hispanics, and African Americans.

Nutritional Assessment

Obesity and history of weight gain are common findings in type 2 diabetes.

Asking the patient for a dietary recall can help identify poor food choices. Dietary recall can be done by asking the patients to remember what they have eaten in the past 24 – 48 hours or by asking them to keep a food diary.

Nutritional assessment includes measurement of height and weight and calculation of body mass index (BMI).

Assessment of the client's level of physical activity helps evaluate energy expenditure.

The healthcare provider should make note of the daily food patterns and the proportional intake of all major food groups.

Other nutritional assessment items should include:
- Regularity and spacing of meals
- Timing of meals (Does the client eat breakfast? Does the client eat most calories at the end of the day?)
- Methods of food preparation
- Recent blood sugar patterns
- Cultural practices with regard to food and food preparation

Assess Medical Health / Psycho-Socioeconomic Status

General Health History

Components of a general health history include:
- Reason for seeking care
  - Sometimes referred to as "chief complaint"
  - Allows client to state his or her priorities and objectives
- Past health history, including duration of diabetes
- Concurrent medical problems
- Family health history
- Allergies to food and medicine
- Immunizations, such as flu and pneumonia vaccines
- Medications (name, dosage, frequency), including over-the-counter and homeopathic medications
- Nutrition history, such as dietary recall and personal/cultural preferences
- Habits, such as alcohol, tobacco, caffeine and recreational drug use
- Exercise and activity patterns
- Rest and sleep patterns
- Stress level and coping mechanisms
- Social support systems
- Cultural preferences with regard to healthcare practices, family support and food preferences

Medication Assessment

Ask for a complete list of all of the medications the client is currently taking. Alternatively, the client can bring all of his or her current medications to the appointment. Current medication history includes making note of prescription and nonprescription medicines, herbal and homeopathic remedies and vitamins. Patients often forget to include nonprescription medications in their reporting if they are not prompted.

Ask if the client has any known allergies to medication. If the client reports a medication allergy, obtain specific information about the effect of the medication. Be aware that a drug reaction may not be a drug allergy. Sometime patients perceive medication side effects as allergic reactions. Interactions with concurrent medications may also be reported as drug allergies.

Find out what medications the client has used for diabetes in the past. Evaluate if they were effective and how they were tolerated by the client.

Fears Associated with Diabetes

It is important to assess the client for diabetes-related fears, since anxiety and phobias can interfere with treatment adherence and self-care behavior.

Asking clients how they feel about common diabetes-related fears can be helpful in establishing trust and can provide an opportunity to help them deal with anxieties. Observing nonverbal behavior and body language can uncover fears that the client is harboring. If a client resists blood glucose monitoring, he or she may be afraid of blood, needles and/or invasive procedures. If a client is resistant to using insulin or certain medications, he or she may have a fear of hypoglycemia.

Common diabetes-related fears include:
- Fear of blood
- Fear of needles
- Fear of hypoglycemia
- Fear of rotating injection sites
- Fear of complications
- Fear of weight gain

Validated assessment tools for diabetes-related fears are available. These include:
- Fear of Hypoglycemia Survey
- Diabetes Fear of Injecting and Self-Testing Questionnaire
- Fear of Progression to Chronic Disease

Family Dynamics and Social Support

Assessment of social support is important because research shows that active family support improves diabetes outcomes for children and adults alike. Conversely, people who do not have a strong social support system are less motivated to engage in self-care. However, social dynamics can also hinder a person's diabetes self-management if significant others downgrade its importance. Therefore, assessment of social and family dynamics must explore the positive and negative effects of the social environment on the individual.

Assessment of family dynamics can include inviting family members to attend appointments and diabetes education programs with the person who has diabetes. This allows for observation of how family members interact and problem-solve together.

It is important to question clients about their support system. They can be asked who helps them with their diabetes management and what they find most helpful from others. It is also important to explore what barriers others present and how the person with diabetes would like things to be different.

Alcohol Abuse

Alcohol can affect blood sugar and impair the judgment needed for good self-care. It can also be dangerous when used with medications to treat diabetes, such as sulfonylureas, metformin and insulin. When taken with insulin or a sulfonylurea, alcohol can trigger hypoglycemia. If taken with metformin, it can cause lactic acidosis.

Assessment of alcohol abuse can be challenging since many people are inaccurate or dishonest in their reporting due to shame, denial or fear of reprisal from the healthcare provider.

Clients under the influence of alcohol may exhibit staggering gait, slurred speech, irritability and mental confusion. These symptoms are also seen with hypoglycemia.

Excessive alcohol consumption may also mimic ketoacidosis, producing fruity breath, drowsiness and coma.

Assessment of alcohol intake includes asking the client how much he or she drinks. This can include asking about how much is consumed in a typical week and the largest amount consumed at one time. Since increased tolerance is a sign of addiction, it is important to ask how much the person needs to become intoxicated.

Tobacco Use

The client who has no intention of quitting tobacco use in the next six months is in the *precontemplation* stage of change. The role of the healthcare provider is to explore feelings and attitudes that may be hindering change.

The client who is aware of the problem and intends to change within the next six months is in the *contemplation stage*. The healthcare provider can encourage behavior change and provide information and resources to help the client.

The client who has started planning for change and will take action within the next month is in the *preparation stage*. The role of the healthcare provider is to facilitate movement toward change with resources and support.

The client who has quit tobacco within the last six months is in the *action stage*. The provider can help the client set short-term goals and solve problems as they arise.

If the client has quit tobacco and maintained the change for six months or more, he or she is in the *maintenance stage*. The provider can offer encouragement and support for the client's success.

Screening for Depression

While depression is a common problem in the general population, its incidence is roughly three times higher among people with diabetes. It is estimated that depression affects 15 – 20% of people with diabetes.

Depression can cause impairment in personal, social and occupational functioning and can significantly affect the self-care behaviors necessary for diabetes management.

Depression is a condition in which the person experiences persistent feelings of sadness and/or a lack of pleasure or interest in almost all activities. Other symptoms may include feelings of guilt or worthlessness, sleep disturbance, low energy, hopelessness and difficulty making decisions.

Educators can screen for depression informally by asking clients if they are experiencing a cluster of symptoms suggestive of depression. There are also validated assessment tools for depression screening. The Beck Depression Inventory (BDI) is a commonly used depression screening tool.

Family of a Child with Diabetes

Determine the normal developmental level of the child. Assess if diabetes is interfering with the child's age-appropriate tasks. Ascertain if the child is at a developmental level appropriate for performing self-care procedures such as checking blood sugar or administering an insulin injection.

Identify how the tasks of diabetes management are distributed. Ask who is responsible for each of the management areas and at what times. Studies indicate that the child is at risk for poor glycemic control when there is disagreement among family members with regard to the delegation of these tasks.

The psychological response of family to diagnosis should be explored. Anxiety and depression are common in parents, especially in the first year after diagnosis. Other common reactions are parental guilt and anger toward the child. Parents may also be fearful of hypoglycemia and the child's risk for long-term complications.

Other assessment data includes:
- Family's understanding of diabetes diagnosis, significance and treatment
- Parents' perceptions of child's ability to participate in diabetes management
- Child's eating habits
- Child's activity patterns
- Child's social adjustment to diabetes (i.e., affect on peer relationships and activities)
- Immunizations

Toddler with Diabetes

Naps and other sleep patterns may interfere with regular feedings. Nighttime feedings are often required to prevent nocturnal hypoglycemia.

Normal toddler behaviors, such as defiance, can increase the challenges of checking blood sugar, taking insulin and eating properly. Assessment should include an exploration of how the parents negotiate these behaviors.

Toddlers often have erratic eating patterns and specific food preferences. They usually require three meals and at least three snacks per day. The timing of eating is important for a child using insulin.

Activity level can be sporadic. Frequent rest periods are counteracted by bursts of intense activity. Extra snacks may be needed to prevent hypoglycemia.

Toddlers are at a high risk for dehydration. Assessment of a parent's ability to prevent, detect and respond to this is important.

Toddlers may not be able to detect hypoglycemia. Toddlers may exhibit hypoglycemia with staggering gait, uncoordinated movements or inactivity. Parents of toddlers may have to test blood sugar frequently to detect hypoglycemia since normal toddler behaviors, such as irritability or defiance, may mask hypoglycemic symptoms.

Adolescent Development

Puberty can be delayed due to poor glycemic control. Physical characteristics of puberty onset are:
- Girls – breast buds, pubic hair, menses (normally at 10 – 11 years of age)
- Boys – pubic hair, enlargement of testicles (normally at age 12 – 16 years)

Due to hormonal changes of puberty, glycemic control deteriorates during this time, even with higher insulin doses.

Psychosocial issues of adolescence include:
- Independence from parents
- Increased awareness of body image
- Increased importance of peer group
- More challenges within the parent-child relationship
- More risk-taking behavior
- Increased sexual awareness and development of sexual relationships

An adolescent with diabetes may struggle more with body image issues related to checking blood sugar, using insulin and being labeled as "a diabetic."

Risk-taking behavior may interfere with good self-care practices.

Independence may be hampered by parents wanting or needing to remain actively involved in diabetes management.

Pregnancy prevention is of utmost importance and the elevated risks of unplanned pregnancy in diabetes must be discussed.

Self-Management in the Older Adult

Functional limitations in the elderly that may affect diabetes self-management may include hearing loss, loss of vision, decline in mobility and cognitive decline. Other challenges may include chronic illness, depression, economic hardship and lack of social support.

Assessment of functional status includes assessing fine motor skills. This includes observing the client's ability to open pill bottles, use a blood glucose meter and draw insulin into a syringe. Other functional motor skills to assess are the person's ability to move around, shop and prepare meals.

Assessment of cognitive status includes orientation, memory and recall. While older people can still learn, the ability to assimilate new information takes longer. Information should be presented in a paced or step-wise fashion. Verbal feedback from the client and return demonstration of skills will assess comprehension.

Economic hardship can result in the inability to purchase proper food or medical supplies or to pay for increasing medical bills. Income and resources must be assessed and the client should be connected to community resources whenever possible.

Overcoming Language Barriers

Body language is often universal. Voice quality, tone, facial expression and mannerisms all communicate something to the client. The educator should keep voice tone friendly, smile appropriately and create a relaxed environment for the client.

The client should be addressed by name and the educator should introduce him or herself. The voice should be kept at normal tone and volume. Talking loud may be perceived as shouting.

Pictorials and visual aids are very helpful in overcoming language barriers. Printed word resources in many different languages are available online. Medical phrase books are also available in many languages.

It is best to simplify the material and use one-syllable, common words. Discuss one topic at a time and use short sentences. Gesture and pantomime where appropriate.

Make use of any translator services available. Be aware of family members as translators. They may pass on their own interpretation of the material, leaving out information they do not want their family member to hear or adding something that they believe should be included.

Behavioral Cues That Indicate That a Client Does Not Understand Teaching
Lack of effective communication may be exhibited by certain nonverbal cues on the part of the client. The client may be nonresponsive when a question is asked. Conversely, he or she may ask questions off topic or about something that was already covered. Attempts to change the subject may also signify that the client does not understand the current topic and is attempting to switch to something more understandable.

Clients who do not understand due to a language barrier may also demonstrate lack of participation or engagement in the teaching session. They may close their eyes, sit passively or fail to ask any questions.

Clients who demonstrate inappropriate laughter or jesting may be trying to cover embarrassment about not understanding the language. On the other hand, a blank expression can also mean that the material is not being communicated. It is important to realize, however, that certain cultures, such as some Asians and Native Americans, perceive direct eye contact as impolite.

Monofilament to Assess Lower Extremities

The American Diabetes Association recommends a thorough foot exam by a healthcare provider at least once a year. This includes testing for loss of protective sensation (LOPS) with a 10-gram monofilament.

This noninvasive procedure uses a flexible bristle to touch the sole, or plantar surfaces of the feet, testing the client's ability to detect injury to the foot. People who cannot feel the monofilament are at higher risk for undetected foot injury and amputation.

The procedure involves having the client remove shoes and socks and sitting with eyes closed. The provider touches the plantar surface of each foot in several spots and asks the client to indicate each time the monofilament is felt.

If the client does not feel the monofilament, he or she is at increased risk for serious foot problems. This client should be counseled on good foot care practices including checking his or her own feet each day for injury.

Assessment of the Diabetic Foot

According to the American Diabetes Association, the components of a complete foot assessment include:
- Inspection for injury, skin breakdown, fungal infections, blisters, red marks from ill-fitting shoes, deformities, dryness or cracking and condition of the toenails.
- Assessment of foot pulses and other signs of circulation.
- Testing for loss of protective sensation (LOPS) with a monofilament and by assessing any one of the following:
  - vibration sensation
  - pinprick sensation
  - ankle reflexes
  - vibration perception threshold

Foot assessment should also include screening for peripheral artery disease, determining history of intermittent claudication and possibly performing an ankle-brachial index.

History should include asking about high-risk conditions for amputation, including:
- Tobacco use
- Previous foot ulcer or amputation
- Neuropathic symptoms
- Visual impairment
- Poor glycemic control

Ankle Brachial Index

The ankle brachial index (ABI) is a test for peripheral artery disease (PAD). Peripheral artery disease is a serious condition that is common in people with diabetes and is often asymptomatic.

Clients with symptoms of PAD, such as intermittent claudication, should have a diagnostic ABI. Intermittent claudication is described as lower extremity pain that occurs during physical activity such as walking and subsides with rest. Other criteria for performing an ABI on people with diabetes include age over 50, smoking, hypertension, dyslipidemia, or diabetes duration of more than 10 years.

The ABI measures blood pressure in the ankle and at the arm while the client is at rest, and then is repeated 5 minutes after walking on a treadmill. Ankle pressure is measured using a standard cuff placed around the calf and a Doppler. Normally, the pressure at both areas should be approximately the same. In PAD, ankle pressures are lower than arm pressures, indicating narrowing of the arteries.

Insulin Injection Sites

The client's insulin injection technique should be reviewed periodically. Clients should understand the importance of proper site selection and rotation. Site rotation prevents hypertrophy, a thickening of the fatty tissue that results from overuse of the same site.

Injection site assessment includes inspection for signs and symptoms of infection such as puffiness or redness. Excessive bruising may indicate bleeding disorder or improper injection technique.

Redness may indicate that the client is using impure insulin or is sensitive to something, such as latex or an additive to the insulin. Insulin allergies are rare with the use of human insulin, which are highly purified. Rotating sites also reduces local irritation.

Tissue atrophy can result from impure insulin and appears as a pitting of the fatty tissue at the injection site. This problem has become less common with the use of human insulin.

Acanthosis Nigricans

Acanthosis nigricans is a skin condition that occurs in up to 90% of children with type 2 diabetes. It is an indicator of hyperinsulinemia and insulin resistance. Acanthosis nigricans is most commonly found in obese dark-skinned children, occurring about 25% more frequently in African American children.

Acanthosis nigricans is characterized by raised, dark brownish to black patches that are velvety to the touch. It most commonly occurs on the back of the neck and other body folds. It can occur at other areas of increased body friction, such as knees and elbows. It can sometimes appear as ring around the neck. Parents or caregivers may mistake the dark coloration for dirt or poor body hygiene and may try to scrub it off.

The condition usually resolves when the underlying insulin resistance is addressed.

Differences in Blood Glucose Monitoring Results

Whole blood consists of plasma, red blood cells, white blood cells and platelets. The blood glucose level of whole blood is lower than the blood glucose of plasma.

Laboratory tests of blood glucose measure glucose in the plasma only, as it can be separated out in the laboratory.

For home blood testing, a drop of whole blood is always used. However, most meters are programmed to calibrate results to conform to plasma values. This allows for better comparison between laboratory and home results. A meter that is programmed to report results as plasma values will be closer to results reported from a laboratory test.

However, some meters still report results as a whole blood measurement. In this case, results of home glucose monitoring will be lower than if a plasma-calibrated meter had been used. The results of whole blood testing are about 10 – 15% lower than results of plasma glucose.

Current Knowledge and Practices

Client's Insulin Injection Technique

Assess patient adherence to the following procedures:
- Washes hands before starting.
- Checks insulin vial for type, expiration date and ensures that the insulin is free of sediment, frosting or other signs of contamination.
- Cleanses top of insulin vial with alcohol.
- Injects air into the insulin vial equal to the amount of insulin to be injected.
- Measures and draws the appropriate amount of insulin.
- Selects appropriate site for subcutaneous injection and has a site rotation system.
- Administers injection subcutaneously. For most people, this involves lightly grasping a fold of skin and injecting at a 90-degree angle. If very thin, the client should inject at a 45-degree angle.
- Follows appropriate technique for disposing of sharps waste.

Troubleshoot Self-Monitored Blood Glucose Results

A comprehensive analysis of factors affecting blood glucose includes:

Food
What did I eat?
How much?
When?
The client should pay particular attention to the amount and type of carbohydrate consumed.

Exercise
How much exercise or physical activity have I had?
Was it more or less than usual?
The client should understand that the blood glucose lowering effects of exercise can be immediate or prolonged, affecting blood glucose for a period of up to 48 or more hours.

Medication
When did I take my diabetes medication (including insulin)?
Did I take it at the right time in relation to meals?
Did I take the correct dose?
Did I properly prepare my insulin (i.e., by rolling the vial of NPH insulin)?
Is my medication expired?

Stress
Am I under a lot of emotional stress?
Am I ill?
Do I have an infected sore?

Blood Glucose Testing
Did I perform the procedure correctly?
Is my meter coded correctly?
Are my test strips expired or damaged?

Carbohydrate Intake

Assess the client's understanding that carbohydrate is the type of food with the greatest effect on postprandial blood glucose levels.

Ask the client to give examples of carbohydrates foods, ensuring that starch, sugar and sweet foods, fruit and milk are all included.

Ensure that the client understands that healthy carbohydrates such as whole grain, fat-free or low-fat dairy products, fruits and vegetables should not be eliminated from the diet due to concerns about their effect on blood glucose.

Assess if the client is consuming a consistent amount of carbohydrate from day to day.

Check to see if the client understands the appropriate amount of carbohydrate that he or she should consume at each meal and each snack.

Review records of blood glucose monitoring and food diaries to assess the effect of carbohydrate choices and portion sizes.

Diet and Lifestyle Changes

Lifestyle changes include medical nutrition therapy, exercise and stress management. The effects of lifestyle changes are usually evaluated at 6 weeks to 3 months following implementation. If blood glucose targets have not been achieved by this time, further changes in nutritional therapy and/or the addition of medication to the regimen are needed.

Educators should avoid the words "diet failure" as the client may interpret this as a personal failure when, in fact, there may be a physiologic need for medication.

As diabetes is a progressive disorder, it is expected that therapy will intensify over time as beta cell function declines. Therefore, evaluation of the therapeutic regimen is ongoing.

Food Diary

The food diary is a record kept by the client of everything that he or she eats in a given period of time. It should include the foods eaten, the approximate amounts, time of day and the situation in which eating occurred. It can be kept for any specified amount of time such as one full week, one day each week, a few days a month or a longer amount of time. A complete food diary will also include a record of exercise.

The food diary helps evaluate food choices and identify where changes are needed. It is also very useful in correlating blood glucose results with food intake. Issues that can be identified by a food diary include inconsistent eating patterns, inappropriate portion sizes, undesirable food choices and amount of carbohydrate consumed. Recording the circumstances under which a person eats raises awareness of unconscious consumption and eating to fulfill emotional needs. For those who have already begun medical nutrition therapy, diaries help evaluate the client's progress toward making the recommended changes.

Type 1 Nutritional Practices

Since people with type 1 diabetes depend upon exogenous insulin, the consumed carbohydrate must closely match insulin dosing.

For those on a fixed insulin dose regimen, consistency in carbohydrate consumption is important. Assess regularity of meals and consistency of carbohydrate portions from day to day.

For clients who adjust their pre-meal insulin doses or use a pump, the educator should assess their understanding and application of the prescribed carbohydrate-to-insulin ratio. A common carbohydrate-to-insulin ratio is 15:1, meaning that the client injects 1 unit of rapid or short-acting insulin for each 15 grams of carbohydrate to be consumed. Provide practice exercises to assess client's ability to adjust insulin dose for different situations such as a large meal, a special party or a late dinner.

Clients with type 1 diabetes are at a higher risk for hypoglycemia. The educator should periodically assess the client's understanding of its prevention and treatment. This includes ensuring that the client is aware that a carbohydrate snack may be needed prior to exercise.

Insulin Adjustment during Exercise

Ensure that clients who use insulin understand that they are at significant risk for exercise-induced hypoglycemia. Hypoglycemia can occur during exercise, immediately after exercise or after a longer period of time. It is important to assess their knowledge and practices with making insulin adjustments for exercise.

Questions to ask include:
- Do you reduce rapid or short-acting insulin prior to exercise? If so, by how much?
  - Reducing by 30 – 50% effectively decreases risk of hypoglycemia.
- Do you reduce intermediate-acting insulin when you are planning to exercise? If so, by how much?
  - Reducing by 10% is recommended.
- Do you check your blood glucose before and after exercise?
  - Provides feedback on results of insulin adjustment and can signal when blood glucose is becoming too low.

Also assess insulin injection technique, ensuring that injections are subcutaneous, not intramuscular.

Safety Precautions Related to Exercise

Clients who use insulin and sulfonylurea medication should know that they are at substantial risk for hypoglycemia. Those using insulin should be aware of how to adjust insulin prior to planned exercise. They should also know how to increase carbohydrate intake at times of unplanned exercise. All clients at risk for hypoglycemia should check blood glucose prior to exercise and carry a fast-acting source of carbohydrate during activity.

Assess clients' adherence to recommendations for using proper footwear and understanding the importance of hydration.

Ensure that clients know to avoid vigorous exercise in hot, humid conditions and when air quality is poor.

Clients who use a beta blocker should know that this medication can impair awareness of hypoglycemia and that they should take special precautions to monitor for it and to prevent it.

Intensity of Exercise

For best results, exercise intensity should be 60 – 85% of the client's age-adjusted heart rate. A precise target heart rate can be calculated from the results of an exercise stress test. Alternatively, the following equation can be used to estimate age-adjusted heart rate:

$$220 - \text{Client's age} = \text{estimated age-adjusted heart rate}$$

The *Rating of Perceived Exertion (RPE)* can also be used to assess exercise intensity. This is a subjective measure in which the client rates how intense the exercise feels on a scale of 0 – 10. Zero means there is no effort at all and 10 corresponds with extremely strong or maximal feelings of exertion. An exertion level of 2 (weak) to 5 (strong) is recommended, depending upon the fitness level of the individual.

Accuracy of a Blood Glucose Meter

According to the American Diabetes Association, blood glucose meters should have total error of 10% or less for blood glucose levels of 30 – 400 mg/dl, 100% of the time.

When the accuracy of the meter is in question, assessment can be done by comparing meter results with laboratory values using the following procedure:
- Meter accuracy should be checked against laboratory values, not against another meter.
- The laboratory test used for comparison should be a fasting plasma glucose test.
- The laboratory test and the meter test should be performed at the same time.
- The test done using the meter should use capillary blood collected from the fingertip or alternate puncture site. A drop of blood from the venous sample should not be placed on the meter strip.
- The venous blood collected in the laboratory should be spun in the centrifuge within 30 minutes of collection.

It should be noted that meters reporting whole blood results will give a reading 11 - 15% lower than the plasma levels measured in the laboratory.

Self-Monitoring of Blood Glucose

The most common source of user error in SMBG is failure to obtain an adequate blood sample. Take every opportunity to assess clients' ability to obtain adequate sample; always ensure proper placement on the test strip. Educators should be familiar with the type of meter and strip system that the client is using, as different systems require different amounts of blood and different blood drop placement technique.

Assess client's procedure for collecting an adequate blood sample. This should include:
- Using warm water to wash hands.
- Dangling or shaking hand below the waist for approximately 30 seconds.
- Setting the adjustable end cap on the lancing device to an appropriate puncture depth.
- Using the "milking" technique to push blood to the fingertip. This involves pushing the blood from the base of the finger to the tip, which is more effective than just squeezing the fingertip.

User Error in Self-Monitoring for Blood Glucose

Failure to obtain an adequate blood sample is the most common source of user error. Assess the client's technique for pricking finger, or alternate site, and ensure proper placement of the blood drop on the test strip.

Defective test strips can lead to inaccurate results. The client should check expiration date before each use, keep reagent vial tightly capped between uses and perform periodic control tests of strips. Strips should also be stored away from extreme heat, cold or humidity.

Clients using certain types of meters should know how to properly calibrate the meter using an inserted strip or setting a code number.

Some older meters use a reflective technology to read blood glucose. These types of meters need to be cleaned if the optic window becomes soiled. Assess the client's ability to properly clean this type of meter according to manufacturer instructions.

Ketones

Ketones can be measured with a home monitoring system that detects ketones in the blood or with dipsticks that test for ketones in the urine.

People with type 1 diabetes are more prone to ketosis than those with type 2 diabetes. These clients should test for ketones whenever blood glucose is persistently elevated over 300 mg/dl. They should also monitor for ketones when they are on a weight reduction diet or when ill, especially with febrile illness of infectious process.

Clients with type 2 diabetes should monitor for ketones during illness or when an infection is present. It is also recommended that they monitor regularly when they are on hypocaloric weight loss diets.

Some pregnant clients with diabetes should monitor for ketones daily, especially if inappropriate calorie restriction is suspected. Pregnant clients should also check for ketones when ill, undergoing severe stress or significantly increasing physical activity.

Clients' Recordkeeping of Self-Monitoring of Blood Glucose

Good recordkeeping is an essential first step in utilizing this important self-management tool.

Although most blood glucose testing meters have an electronic memory function, written records of SMBG should also be kept on paper. Instruct clients that the electronic memory is an optional convenience for use in writing down results at a later time.

Clients can keep effective records in printed logbooks, on computer spreadsheets or on notebook paper. A chart fashioned in lines and columns, indicating blood glucose results corresponding to specific times of day, helps identify patterns. Patterns can then be used to adjust food, exercise or medication. Clients should distinguish between pre-meal and postprandial results to help interpret the effect of food on blood glucose. They can also keep notes of foods eaten, medications taken and exercise patterns.

Some clients may prefer to record results as a graph or download graphs of their blood glucose using computer programs. This is an acceptable alternative method of recordkeeping.

Client Medication Adherence

Is the medication taken on a regular schedule?

Does the client know the right time to take the medication? For example, glipizide works best when taken 30 minutes before the meal. Other medications, such as metformin are best taken with food to reduce gastrointestinal upset. Statin medications are most effective when taken at bedtime.

What does the client do if he or she misses a dose? The client should know not to double the dose of medication when a dose is missed.

Is the client taking the dose that was prescribed?

Is the client up to date on laboratory testing of liver and kidney function, as appropriate?

If using a sulfonylurea or insulin, what is the client's eating pattern and spacing of meals? Meals should be no more than 4 – 5 hours apart to prevent hypoglycemia.

What does the client do when blood sugar is low (if applicable)?

Insurance

Medicare Benefit
Medicare is the largest federally funded payer of health insurance coverage.

Eligibility criteria include:
- Age over 65
- Disabled, any age
- End-stage renal disease, any age

Parts of Medicare include:
- Medicare Part A covers hospital, skilled nursing, home health or hospice. Beneficiary pays deductible.
- Medicare Part B covers physician office visits, outpatient services, laboratory costs, equipment and supplies. Part B is elective and the beneficiary pays the premiums.
- Medicare Part C, also known as Medicare Advantage, covers things not covered by Parts A and B, such as extra days in the hospital. Although not available in all areas, Part C provides an option for some to avoid purchasing "MediGap" insurance to fill gaps in Medicare coverage. Beneficiary pays a monthly premium.

- Medicare Part D is prescription drug insurance that lowers the cost of medications. Beneficiaries pay a monthly premium and choose a drug plan from a participating private company.

Fee-for-Service and Managed Care Health Insurance Plans
Fee-for-service plans, also known as indemnity plans, reimburse the beneficiary after medical expenses have been incurred. Claim forms are typically utilized. The insured usually pays an annual deductible amount for the first expenses incurred during the calendar year. Once the deductible is satisfied, the insurer pays a percentage, often 80%, of the incurred expenses. Indemnity plans offer the consumer free choice of healthcare provider.

Managed care plans are administered by health maintenance organizations (HMOs). They generally require lower premiums because they have greater cost control. Members pay a nominal copayment for services rendered and there are no claim forms or annual deductibles. Managed care plans are more restrictive in choice of provider and some HMOs are provider-owned. This type of plan places more emphasis on preventive services.

Fee-for-service and managed care plans represent two extremes in health insurance coverage. In between, there are other types of plans such as preferred provider organizations (PPOs) and managed fee-for-service plans.

Federal Insurance Programs
Medicare – Provides full medical services to people age 65 and older, people permanently disabled of any age and all people with end stage renal disease.

Veterans Administration (VA) – Care is provided free of charge to veterans who have service-related medical conditions, served in specific wars or meet low-income criteria. Veterans not meeting these criteria can also receive medical care with copayments.

Indian Health Services (IHS) – Medical services are provided free of charge to American Indians and Alaska Natives who are members of federally recognized tribes.

TRICARE – Offers healthcare services to active duty and retired military, their families and their survivors.

Bureau of Primary Health Care – Provides medical services to vulnerable, underserved people having geographic, financial or cultural barriers to health care. Eligible beneficiaries pay on sliding scale basis at federally qualified centers, many of them in rural areas.

<u>"Conditions of Coverage"</u>

Eligibility – Includes membership criteria, such as age in the case of Medicare, or being a being a policyholder under private insurance plans. Other eligibility criteria may include being classified in a diagnostic group or requiring a specific type of medical treatment.

Covered benefits – These are the types of services and supplies that the insurance plan covers. Examples of covered benefits may include laboratory services, specific procedures, equipment such as glucose monitors, and medical supplies. The insurers normally have specific criteria under which payment for covered services will be rendered. For example, a carrier may only pay for a specific brand of glucose meter and may stipulate the quantity of testing strips that can be distributed over a specified period of time.

Exclusions – These are items not covered by the insurance plan. Common exclusions are eyeglasses, dentistry and cosmetic surgery.

Medical necessity – Certain criteria must be met and documentation provided to justify that the services or supplies are necessary.

Intervention

Collaborate with Patient / Family

Individualizing a Diabetes Education Plan

Because people with diabetes are a heterogeneous group, educational programs should be relevant to the individuals being served. This involves tailoring the program content to meet the characteristics of the learner while recognizing that participants have the right and responsibility to set their own educational and behavioral goals.

All aspects of the educational program, including learning objectives, teaching content, methodology, and communication style, should be personalized. Individualization is considered an appropriate and viable option for both individual and group education programs.

Individual characteristics to consider when developing an individualized teaching plan include:
- Learning styles
- Culture
- Educational level and literacy
- Psychosocial status
- Cognitive status
- Functional limitations
- Readiness to learn and make behavior change
- Baseline knowledge
- Age and developmental level
- Personal and metabolic goals
- Access to resources

<u>Diabetes Education Plan Individualized for an Acutely Ill Patient</u>
Acutely ill patients may be distracted by pain or other types of physical discomfort. The direct effects of the illness or medications may induce lethargy or impair cognitive functioning and memory. Therefore, the teaching plan for these patients should focus on basic "survival skill' information. Assessment of specific problems the patient is having helps prioritize and focus teaching content.

Patient safety should be assessed, and information to promote safety should be considered a priority. This may include such things as medication instruction or the prevention, recognition and treatment of hypoglycemia. Observation of body language can be used to assess patient response and can help determine the amount and type of information the patient is able to assimilate. Involvement of caregivers and family members is important.

Arrangements for follow up with the acutely ill patient are important so education that is more detailed can be provided at a later time.

Learning and Behavioral Objectives

Both learning and behavioral objectives are developed based on individual assessment and in collaboration with the client. Both types of objectives are written as measurable outcomes so that the results of education can be evaluated.

Learning objectives assess knowledge in an indirect way, since learning cannot actually be witnessed. Behavioral objectives are a more direct assessment since behavior is something that can be observed.

The purpose of learning objectives is to spell out the intended content of education. An example of a learning objective is: *Describe the effect of carbohydrate on blood glucose.*

Behavioral objectives provide the client with a plan for taking specific actions that he or she feels have value and are feasible. An example of a behavioral objective is: *Walk for 20 minutes during lunch break 5 days a week for the next 2 weeks.*

Information Presented in a Diabetes Education Program

The empowerment approach to diabetes education recognizes that the person with diabetes holds the primary rights and responsibilities for his or her own self-care. In diabetes education programs, the sequence of information should take into account the priorities of the client.

One of the first messages that participants should hear in a program is that diabetes is a self-managed condition.

Client priorities can be assessed by asking what they would like to learn and by showing a list of possible topics from which to select.

Psychosocial issues should be addressed early in the program. Educators should remember that having diabetes is not an academic exercise, but a situation that affects the daily lives of clients. Therefore, a physiology lesson on diabetes is less important than learning how to eat the right foods.

Another important factor in prioritizing program content is safety. Learning to use insulin or to prevent and manage hypoglycemia are examples of high-priority topics that may need to be covered first when time is limited.

Instructional Methods

Computer as Instructional Method
Computer programs and online resources are appropriate choices for self-directed learners and those who are comfortable with technology. While many older adults are proficient in the use of the computer, lack of experience or functional limitations may make this an inappropriate choice for some.

People who prefer to learn independently and at their own pace may prefer computerized education. This type of learning often provides the opportunity for interactive learning as well.

Clients with unusual hours, limited time or inflexible schedules may benefit from the 24 hour access provided by computers.

Clients of lower socioeconomic status may not own a computer. Computers are available for public use at most public libraries, though the time one is allowed to remain at the computer is limited.

Clients who consult internet sites for information on diabetes self-management should be cautioned that not all sources of information are reliable. Sites hosted by major authoritative bodies, such as the American Diabetes Association, or by government bodies and universities are usually most appropriate.

Group Discussion as Instructional Method

Group discussion supports the empowerment approach to diabetes education by allowing participants to direct the content of education and practice decision-making in a supportive environment. This methodology allows clients to seek and acquire the information that is most important to them. The role of the educator in the discussion group is to provide guidance and support and to keep exchange focused on learning objectives and within time constraints.

Group discussion is an appropriate methodology for adult learners as it is an active, self-directed approach that is relevant to the individual. An example of an appropriate topic for group discussion would be to share blood glucose logs and share suggestions for how to interpret and respond to results.

A limitation of group discussions is that the educator has less control over program content than in traditional lecture programs. Also, some group members may monopolize, leaving others with unmet needs. Clients with impaired hearing or language barriers may not be appropriate for group discussions.

Demonstration as Instructional Method

Demonstration as an instructional method allows for an active hands-on learning experience. It is appropriate for teaching diabetes self-management skills such as using a monitor to test blood glucose, drawing and injecting insulin and calculating insulin dosages.

Demonstration has the benefit of allowing the educator to directly observe behaviors that can indicate learning has taken place. Likewise, it can help identify areas that require additional instruction.

A limitation of demonstration is that it can be difficult to do effectively in large groups, as participants may not be able to see the instructor's demonstration and the instructor may not be able to observe a return demonstration by each member. Demonstration can also be a more time-consuming instructional method.

Role Playing As Instructional Method

Role playing is an interactive teaching methodology appropriate for a variety of age groups, including children, teens and adults. It provides the opportunity to practice problem-solving, explore feelings and practice new behaviors. It can be equally effective in both individual and group education programs.

Appropriate topics for role playing would be to practice asking for support from significant others or learning to respond assertively to peers who ask questions about having diabetes or using insulin.

Facilitating effective role plays requires skill on the part of the educator. Some people may not be comfortable being asked to "act" and should be allowed to be an observer. Assessment of hearing, language and culture are all important before deciding to implement role playing as an instructional method.

Group Teaching Content and Methods

Reading, writing, listening, watching and doing are examples of preferred learning styles. Many people have a combination of preferred learning styles.

Literacy includes the level at which one reads and writes, as well as the ability to speak, compute and solve problems.

Group classes usually include people with varying learning styles and degrees of literacy. To meet a wider variety of needs, instructional methods should include a variety of formats. Videotapes are an example of a format that appeals to a wide variety of learners. Group discussions and role-plays are also appropriate for heterogeneous groups, as clients can learn through problem-solving and brainstorming with others who have diabetes.

Reading materials written at a lower reading level are often preferred by clients regardless of their literacy or educational level.

Instructional Methods for Various Age Groups

Preschool children learn best from simple question and answer sessions based on age-appropriate experiences. Props, such as puppets and dolls, are often used to appeal to the child's developmental level.

School-aged children learn best through games and puzzles as well as age-appropriate videos and interactive computer programs.

Teens are motivated by peer influence. Therefore, same-age group classes and discussions are most appropriate. At this age, learning to make decisions and solve problems are important components of diabetes education. Diabetes camps can be very valuable learning experiences for this age group.

Adults prefer learning content that is relevant to their day-to-day living. Practical content that addresses everyday problems is most appropriate for adults. Adults also prefer self-directed learning. Therefore, collaboration on the educational objectives is appropriate with this population.

Setting Behavioral Goals

Behavioral goals for diabetes education are based upon an individualized assessment of client needs. They are based on knowledge gaps identified during assessment and on identified client preferences.

Behavioral goals are developed in collaboration with the client, with the client initiating the direction of the goals. Collaboration with the multidisciplinary team provides the information and guidance needed for informed decision-making on the part of the client.

Tools that the educator can use to help facilitate goal setting include behavioral change theory, the patient empowerment approach and patient-centered communication.

A self-directed approach to goal setting empowers clients and keeps them involved in the learning process. In addition to providing information for informed decision-making, the educator's role in goal setting includes promoting confidence or self-efficacy, facilitating effective problem-solving, developing coping skills and identifying strategies to overcome barriers.

Finally, goals should include metrics for success that are developed in collaboration with the client.

"SMART" Behavioral Goals

Behavioral goals should be individualized and developed in collaboration with the client. They represent a planned change in behavior that reflects the values of the client. In order to be successful, the clients should select goals that they feel will reap benefit, that they are interested in doing and that they are able to do.

The acronym "SMART" is often used in developing behavioral goals.

S – Specific – Tells *what* the person will do.
M – Measurable – Tells *how much, how often and/or how many.*
A – Achievable – Is something the person wants to do and can commit to.
R – Realistic – The person feels confident that they can do what they have planned.
T – Time bound – Specifies the time period after which the behavior will be evaluated.

An example of a SMART goal:

I will check my blood sugar twice a day, every day, before breakfast and before dinner for 2 weeks.

Teach / Counsel Principles of Diabetic Care

Type 1 Diabetes

Characteristics of type 1 diabetes include:
- Results from autoimmune destruction of the beta cells of the pancreas.
- Leads to an absolute deficiency of endogenous insulin.
- Usually involves rapid destruction of beta cells in children and slower destruction in adults.
- Children and adolescents sometimes present with ketoacidosis as the first sign of the disease.
- Absence of endogenous insulin secretion is manifested by low C-peptide levels.
- Causes include genetic predisposition and environmental factors.
- Patients are usually lean, but normal or overweight status does not preclude diagnosis.
- Patients are also prone to Hashimoto's thyroiditis, Addison's disease, vitiligo, celiac sprue, autoimmune hepatitis, pernicious anemia and myasthenia gravis.

Type 2 Diabetes

Characteristics of type 2 diabetes include:
- Pathophysiology involves insulin resistance and relative insulin deficiency.
- Treatment with exogenous insulin is not needed for immediate survival.
- Unlike type 1 diabetes, there is no autoimmune destruction of pancreatic beta cells.
- Obesity or increased body fat in abdominal region increases the risk.
- Ketoacidosis is rare.
- Often goes undetected for years.
- Hyperglycemia develops gradually in earlier stages of disease and is usually asymptomatic.
- Occurs with higher incidence in people having hypertension and dyslipidemia.
- Risk factors include increased age, obesity, sedentary lifestyle, positive family history and personal history of gestational diabetes.
- Genetic predisposition is a significant risk factor.

Pancreatic Beta Cell Destruction

Genetic defects of beta cells lead to maturity onset diabetes of the young (MODY), manifested by the onset of hyperglycemia in people usually younger than age 25.

Genetic defects of insulin action result in abnormalities of the insulin receptors, leading to insulin resistance and hyperglycemia.

Diseases, conditions and events that can lead to the onset of diabetes include pancreatitis, trauma, infection, cancer, hemochromatosis and cystic fibrosis.

Excessive production of hormones that are antagonistic to insulin can cause diabetes. These hormones include growth hormone, cortisol, glucagons and epinephrine.

Drugs that can impair insulin secretion and precipitate diabetes in insulin-resistant people include nicotinic acid, glucocorticoids, alpha-interferon, thiazides and Dilantin.

Viral infections such as congenital rubella, coxsackievirus B, cytomegalovirus and mumps have been known to induce diabetes.

Other genetic syndromes associated with diabetes onset include Down syndrome, Klinefelter syndrome and Turner syndrome.

Increased Risk for Diabetes

Impaired fasting glucose (IFG) and impaired glucose tolerance (IGT) are categories of increased risk for diabetes collectively known as "Prediabetes." They represent an intermediate category where blood glucose levels are elevated above normal, but not high enough to be classified as diabetes. Both conditions are associated with obesity, increased abdominal fat, dyslipidemia and hypertension.

The American Diabetes Association stipulates that these are not true diagnostic categories, but represent a condition of elevated risk for the development of both diabetes and cardiovascular disease.

IFG is characterized by fasting plasma glucose levels of 100 mg/dl – 125 mg/dl.

IGT is manifested by 2-hour oral glucose tolerance test values of 140 mg/dl – 199 mg/dl.

In 2010, the American Diabetes Association recommended that an A1C level of 5.7 – 6.4% be used as an additional criterion for identifying increased risk for diabetes.

Diagnosis of Diabetes

According to the American Diabetes Association, diabetes is diagnosed if any of the following criteria are met:
- A1C ≥ 6.5%   OR
- Fasting plasma glucose (FPG) ≥ 126 mg/dl.
  Fasting means no caloric intake for 8 or more hours.   OR
- 2-hour plasma glucose ≥ 200 mg/dl during an oral glucose tolerance test (OGTT).
  The test should be performed using a glucose load of 75 grams and performed as described by the World Health Organization.   OR
- Random plasma glucose ≥ 200 mg/dl when patient presents with classic symptoms of hyperglycemia, such as polydipsia and polyuria.

If the presence of hyperglycemia is not unequivocal on the A1C, FPG or OGGT, repeat testing is indicated.

ADA Testing for Type 2 in Children

Children who are overweight and have any TWO of the risk factors listed below should be tested for type 2 diabetes, beginning at age 10 or at onset of puberty if puberty occurs at an earlier age.

Risk factors:
- Family history of type 2 diabetes in first- or second-degree relatives
- Native American, African American, Hispanic/Latino, Asian American, Pacific Islander

- Signs of insulin resistance, such as acanthosis nigricans, hypertension, dyslipidemia, or polycystic ovary syndrome
- Maternal history of gestational diabetes during child's gestation

Overweight is defined as:
- BMI > 85th percentile for age and sex
- Weight for height > 85th percentile
- Weight > 12 – 30% above ideal

Fasting plasma glucose should be done on children at risk every 3 years.

Modifiable Risk Factors for Diabetes Prevention

Diet – Decreasing calories and total dietary fat, especially saturated fat, is recommended to reduce risk for type 2 diabetes. In addition, increasing the intake of dietary fiber and whole grains is recommended.

Body Weight – Results of the Diabetes Prevention Program (DPP) showed that when high-risk overweight subjects lost 5 – 7% of their initial body weight, risk for developing diabetes was reduced by 58%.

Waist Circumference – Men having waist circumference greater than 40 inches and women with waist circumference greater than 35 inches are at higher risk for diabetes. Waist circumference has been found to be a stronger predictor for diabetes risk than both BMI and body weight.

Sedentary Lifestyle – Exercise boosts both carbohydrate metabolism and insulin sensitivity. The DPP has shown that subjects who participated in approximately 150 minutes of moderate intensity exercise per week, in addition to implementing healthy eating choices, significantly reduced their risk for type 2 diabetes.

Pathophysiology of Type 1 Diabetes

Type 1 diabetes is the result of an autoimmune attack on the beta cells of the pancreas.

Although hyperglycemic symptoms, and even ketoacidosis, may appear abruptly, the disease begins to develop long before it becomes apparent.

While there is a genetic predisposition, many people with genetic risk do not develop the disease. An environmental or viral trigger is believed necessary for the disease to express itself in predisposed individuals.

Islet cell antibodies appear early in the course of type 1 diabetes and direct their attack against the beta cells. While there are several different islet cell antibodies, a high titer of glutamic acid decarboxylase (GAD) is considered the best immunologic predictor for the development of type 1 diabetes.

The onset of illness is usually abrupt, followed by a "honeymoon period" in which beta cells are in a compensatory phase and temporary normoglycemia results. Ultimately, continued beta cell destruction leads to acute loss of glycemic control, resulting in the permanent need for exogenous insulin.

Pathophysiology of Type 2 Diabetes

Relative insulin deficiency – Insulin production by the beta cells of the pancreas is insufficient for the body's needs. There is a 50% reduction in beta cell mass in people with type 2 diabetes.

Insulin resistance – Insulin receptors, found mostly on muscle and liver tissue, have developed a resistance to the biological activity of insulin. Insulin resistance is present years before the onset of hyperglycemia.

Overproduction of glucose by the liver – Normally increased insulin levels in the blood suppress hepatic glucose production. In type 2 diabetes, insulin resistance of hepatic receptors results in continued hepatic glucose production despite circulating insulin levels.

Maturity Onset Diabetes of the Young

MODY is a rare type of secondary diabetes associated with inherited genetic defects on chromosomes 7, 12 and 20. Due to these chromosomal defects, beta cell function is impaired, leading to early onset of mild hyperglycemia. While insulin secretion is impaired, insulin action and sensitivity are unaffected.

Although MODY affects young people, it should not be confused with type 2 diabetes in youth.

Since there is no way to ameliorate the cause of MODY, treatment relies on the traditional cornerstones of therapy for diabetes – medical nutrition therapy, exercise and medication.

Fuel Metabolism

Insulin and Amylin in Fuel Metabolism
Insulin and amylin are both glucoregulatory hormones secreted by the pancreatic beta cells in response to an increase in blood glucose. Initially, they are secreted into the portal vein before being released into the general circulation. They work in a complementary fashion to regulate the arrival and departure of glucose in the blood.

Insulin is taken up by receptors in the peripheral and hepatic tissue, resulting in the transport of glucose from the blood. Insulin also inhibits glucose production from the liver and inhibits the release of glucagon from the alpha cells of the pancreas.

Amylin is secreted along with insulin from the pancreatic beta cells. Like insulin, it inhibits glucagon secretion. It also regulates the appearance of glucose in the blood by slowing gastric emptying and possibly suppressing the appetite.

Normal Fuel Metabolism in the Fasting, Fed and Post-Absorptive States
During the fasting state, blood glucose levels are maintained primarily through hepatic sources. Hepatic sources of glucose include those made by the liver (glyconeogenesis) and those stored in the liver as glycogen, then converted into glucose (glycogenolysis).

When carbohydrate is ingested, circulating glucose increases significantly and phase 1 of fuel metabolism is initiated. In this "fed state," plasma insulin levels are high and insulin acts to transport glucose from the blood. At the same time, glucagon levels are low. Since the main role of glucagon is to stimulate gluconeogenesis by the liver, glucagon activity significantly declines during the fed state.

Phase 2 of fuel metabolism is also known as the post-absorptive state, occurring 4 – 16 hours after food is consumed. During this time, plasma insulin levels decrease as glucagon levels increase. Blood glucose during this time is maintained from hepatic sources.

Blood Glucose Pattern Management

Pattern management is a comprehensive approach to diabetes self-management that is often associated with intensive insulin therapy. However, it can also be useful for identifying any appropriate changes that could be made to improve glycemic control.

Pattern management involves analyzing 3 – 5 days worth of blood glucose readings and identifying patterns of high or low blood glucose that occur at the same time each day. Adjustments can then be made based on a blood glucose trend, rather than responding to a single reading.

Pattern management allows choices in how to respond to these patterns. For example, the insulin or medication doses could be adjusted up or down based on a blood glucose pattern. Other choices would be to increase or decrease carbohydrate consumption or to change exercise frequency, timing or intensity.

Weight Loss for Type 2 Diabetes

There is a strong correlation between overweight or obesity and type 2 diabetes. Much of this is due to an association between excess body fat and insulin resistance. Several major studies have concluded that even a modest amount of weight loss can prevent the development of diabetes in high-risk people.

Weight loss, through healthy eating and exercise, can improve glycemic control and decrease the need for medication in people with type 2 diabetes. On the other hand, progressive loss of beta cell function over time can result in the need for medication despite changes in lifestyle. At minimum, healthy lifestyle choices leading to weight loss improve glycemic control and reduce the risk for cardiovascular disease and a host of other health problems.

Maintaining weight loss can be one of the most challenging aspects of diabetes self-management. Clients can become frustrated and require emotional support as much as education. Correlating weight loss and improved A1C can help boost confidence and motivate patients.

Multiple Medications for Diabetes

As a naturally progressive disorder, diabetes usually requires increasingly intensive therapy over time. This is due to progressive loss of beta cell function and/or increasing insulin resistance.

Various classes of diabetes medications target the different physiological defects of type 2 diabetes. Often, combination therapy, or simultaneously using medications from different classes, is necessary to gain and maintain glycemic control.

In addition to glycemic control, ameliorating the high risk for cardiovascular disease is imperative for good diabetes management. As hypertension and dyslipidemia are often comorbidities with insulin resistance, these usually require their own pharmacological intervention in addition to the medications patients with diabetes may need to achieve and maintain glycemic control.

Due to the complexity of the type 2 diabetes disease process, coupled with the need for cardiovascular protection, polypharmacy is common in the treatment of type 2 diabetes.

Basal Bolus Insulin for Type 1 Diabetes

Basal bolus insulin therapy is designed to mimic the normal patterns of insulin secretion, such as that observed in a person without diabetes.

Basal insulin refers to small amounts of insulin that are secreted continuously. This is sometimes referred to as "background insulin" as it is secreted in steady states and causes no peaks in action.

Bolus insulin refers to bursts of insulin secretion that occur in response to increased blood glucose.

With exogenous insulin therapy, it is possible to closely mimic the normal basal bolus insulin production of the non-diabetic pancreas. The choices for doing this include:
- Continuous subcutaneous insulin infusion (CSII), also known as insulin pump. The pump is programmed to release basal insulin at selected rates. Bolus insulin is controlled by the user each time food is ingested to deliver the calculated insulin-to-carbohydrate ratio.
- Multiple daily injections. This choice involves injecting a long-acting insulin analog at least once or twice a day and possibly several times a day or more to provide basal insulin. The user injects a calculated dose of fast or rapid-acting insulin to cover meals.

Basal Bolus Insulin

Basal bolus insulin therapy is the preferred choice for people with type 1 diabetes because they produce neither basal nor bolus insulin of their own. Using basal insulin reduces hepatic glucose production while bolus insulin limits excursions in post-meal blood glucose. Basal bolus insulin therapy, which is delivered via insulin pump or by multiple daily injections, allows for a more flexible lifestyle and the best possible blood glucose control.

Basal bolus insulin therapy requires the client and provider to have a good understanding of the action times of different insulins. The client must also be able to understand the basal bolus concept and to consistently follow through with this type of regimen. A certain level of math literacy (numeracy) is also needed.

For some clients, premixed insulin such as 70/30 NPH/regular may be desirable. However, this does not allow for as much flexibility in the timing of eating or exercise. It also does not allow for the best possible control of blood glucose.

Amylin Analog

People with insulin deficiency are also amylin deficient. Amylin is a hormone that is normally secreted by the pancreatic beta cells along with insulin. It serves to reduce postprandial hyperglycemia and cause satiety, leading to weight loss.

Pramlintide is an amylin analog given as an injection.

Nausea is a common side effect of pramlintide, but it is usually dose-related and subsides over time.

The potential for insulin-induced hypoglycemia is a major concern with using pramlintide. The insulin dose must therefore be adjusted down when the amylin analog is started. Also, the client must be willing to test blood glucose numerous times a day to monitor and prevent hypoglycemia when using pramlintide.

Insulin for Type 2 Diabetes

The decision to initiate insulin should be based on the need for glycemic control. If lifestyle interventions and oral medications do not achieve control, starting insulin improves the chances for a better outcome. Unfortunately, some patients perceive this as a sign of failure or punishment for not achieving control.

An advantage of insulin therapy is that, as beta cell function naturally declines, the insulin dosage can be adjusted up, with no ceiling, to achieve glycemic goals.

Weight gain when initiating insulin is a concern. Patients can count carbohydrates and increase exercise to offset this risk. Concurrent use of metformin can also help.

Hypoglycemia is a significant risk for patients using insulin. Patients must be taught to closely match the timing and content of meals with their insulin dosing and to be alert for signs of impending hypoglycemia.

Pain, inconvenience and fear of needles are all reasons why patients resist starting insulin. Because of its effectiveness in gaining glycemic control and producing better outcomes, educators must communicate positively about the advantages of insulin.

Self-Monitoring of Blood Glucose and A1C

Recommended target ranges for self-monitoring of blood glucose should be individualized and can vary according to age group. While the gold standard test of glycemic control is the A1C, daily blood glucose values from self-monitoring should correlate with A1C results.

According to the ADA, general target blood glucose goals from self-monitoring for most adults are:

Fasting   90 – 130 mg/dl

Postprandial   Less than 180 mg/dl

Like target ranges for self-monitoring of blood glucose, A1C targets should be individualized. Age, pregnancy status, hypoglycemic awareness and comorbidities are factors to consider when recommending a goal for glycemic control.

In general, the ADA recommends a target A1C of 7% or less for most people. The goal may be less stringent for someone with limited life expectancy or with hypoglycemic unawareness. A more stringent goal may be recommended for a younger person if this can be achieved without significantly increasing the risk for hypoglycemia.

Blood Glucose Targets for Infant through 19 Years

Blood glucose target ranges should be individualized based on assessment of risk and benefit for each patient.

As a general guideline, the ADA recommends:

Ages 0 - 6 100 – 180 mg/dl before meals
      110 – 120 mg/dl bedtime
      A1C 7.5 – 8.5%

Ages 6 - 12 90 – 180 mg/dl before meals
      100 – 180 mg/dl bedtime
      A1C < 8.0%

Ages 13 - 19 90 – 130 mg/dl before meals
      90 – 150 mg/dl bedtime
      A1C < 7.5%

Infants and very young children have more liberal goals to prevent undetected hypoglycemia and protect the developing central nervous system.

Goals for all age groups should be adjusted if the child is having frequent hypoglycemia.

Glycemic Targets for an Elderly Client

Goals for glycemic control should not automatically be raised for elderly clients, as a target A1C of 7% may be appropriate for some people over the age of 65.

However, certain factors related to the aging process do require special consideration when recommending glycemic targets for this population. Reasons to consider more lenient targets for older people may include:
- Impaired functional status
- Poor social support or isolated living situation
- Decline in cognitive function
- Hypoglycemic unawareness
- Decreased life expectancy

Hypoglycemic unawareness is a common change with aging, so choice of medication should take this into account. Selection of medication for elderly clients should also take into account declining kidney and liver function.

Hypertension

Control of blood pressure is considered paramount for the reduction of cardiovascular risk in people with diabetes.

The American Diabetes Association (ADA) recommends a blood pressure goal of less than 130/80 mmHg for people with diabetes.

Therapeutic lifestyle interventions are recommended when blood pressure is between 130/80 mmHg and 139/89 mmHg. Lifestyle modifications include weight loss, exercise, tobacco cessation and limitation of sodium intake.

When the blood pressure is greater than 140/90 mmHg, antihypertensive medication is usually added to therapeutic lifestyle interventions when either the diastolic or systolic value is elevated.

Angiotensin-converting enzyme (ACE) inhibitors or angiotensin receptor blockers are considered first-line pharmacologic therapy for hypertension in people with diabetes.

Lipid Abnormalities

Dyslipidemia associated with type 2 diabetes includes reduced HDL cholesterol and elevated triglyceride levels. These abnormalities, along with hypertension, are known as metabolic syndrome and are associated with increased risk for cardiovascular disease.

Elevated LDL cholesterol is not specifically associated with type 2 diabetes. However, since LDL cholesterol particles are atherogenic and their presence increases cardiovascular risk, this type of cholesterol is also targeted for control in people with diabetes.

The American Diabetes Association (ADA) recommends an LDL cholesterol of less than 100 mg/dl. Further reduction to less than 70 mg/dl is recommended for people with very high risk.

Goals for HDL cholesterol and triglycerides vary among the authoritative bodies.

Lifestyle modifications, such as increased physical activity and a diet low in saturated fat, are recommended for dyslipidemia. Statin medication is recommended when LDL cholesterol is greater than 135 mg/dl if the person has no other cardiovascular risk factors. Statin medication should be started in all patients with diabetes who have increased cardiovascular risk, regardless of baseline lipid levels.

Diabetes Prevention Program

The DPP was a large multicenter study which demonstrated that the onset of diabetes can be prevented or delayed in high-risk subjects when certain lifestyle modifications are implemented. The at-risk population was identified as having glucose intolerance. Many of the participants came from high-risk minority groups.

It was shown that healthy eating and increasing physical activity, which led to weight loss, decreased the risk for developing diabetes by 58%.

Based on the findings from this study, the following recommendations for lifestyle modification are recommended to prevent or delay the onset of type 2 diabetes:
- Weight loss of 5 – 7% of baseline weight
- A diet low in fat and calories but high in fiber
- Moderate exercise for 150 minutes per week

Evaluate Quality Of Life

Quality of life is a somewhat ambiguous term, but there is general agreement that it encompasses the client's subjective appraisal of his or her emotional, psychosocial and physical well-being. Improving quality of life is a primary goal of diabetes self-management education.

Certain aspects of diabetes have been shown to decrease quality of life, such as insulin dependence, retinopathy and comorbid conditions.

There are several diabetes-specific tools for measuring quality of life. These include:
- Diabetes Quality of Life Measure (DQOL)
- Diabetes Treatment Satisfaction Questionnaire
- Diabetes-Specific Quality of Life Scale (DSQOLS)

Examples of domains measured by these tools include:
- Satisfaction with diabetes treatment
- Impact of treatment, such as experience with hypoglycemia and adherence to dietary guidelines
- Impact of diabetes on social, physical and vocational functioning
- Psychological aspects, such as worry about future health

Simply asking the client how diabetes is affecting his or her life is an informal and expedient way to assess quality of life.

A1C Test

The glycated hemoglobin A1c (A1C) test is the gold standard test for measuring glycemic control in people with diabetes. Results of the landmark Diabetes Control and Complications Trial (DCCT) and other major studies have shown that elevated A1C levels are directly related to long-term complications of diabetes.

The A1C provides a depiction of the average blood glucose over the previous 2 – 3 month period. Glucose in the blood attaches to the hemoglobin molecule, which is measured by the A1C test. While recommendations for glycemic control are always individualized, the target A1C for most people is 7% or less.

In 2010, its use a tool for diagnosing diabetes was established by the American Diabetes Association (ADA). An A1C ≥ 6.5% is now an accepted diagnostic criterion for diabetes. The ADA states that in order to be valid, the A1C test must be done by a standardized and certified laboratory method.

Lipid Testing

People with diabetes have a risk for cardiovascular disease that is 2 – 4 times greater than that of the non-diabetic population. This largely due to the metabolic syndrome associated with the insulin resistance of type 2 diabetes and includes dyslipidemia and hypertension.

Because of this elevated cardiovascular risk, lipid testing and treatment of dyslipidemia are paramount to the care and treatment of diabetes.

Fasting lipids should be tested at least annually or every two years if the patient is at low risk. Because the dyslipidemia associated with diabetes includes reduced HDL cholesterol and increased triglycerides, a complete lipid panel is usually warranted.

Renal Function Tests

Microalbuminuria – measured by any of three methods
- Spot urine collection to measure albumin-to-creatinine ratio:
  - Most commonly used of the three options.
  - Normal value is less than 30 mcg/ml.
- 24-hour urine collection to compare simultaneous urine and serum creatinine clearance
- Timed urine collection, such as overnight or for 4 hours

Creatinine clearance – to estimate glomerular filtration rate (GFR)
- Depends upon carefully timed urine sample, usually over 24 hours.
- Inaccuracy in timing or an incomplete sample can lead to erroneous results.
- Provides a direct method of estimating GFR.

Serum creatinine (SCr) – to estimate GFR indirectly
- Can be calculated based on patient age and weight.
- Subtle changes in SCr can herald major loss of renal function.

Blood Urea Nitrogen (BUN) – also to indirectly measure GFR
- Less sensitive marker of early diabetic nephropathy
- Used with SCr to monitor renal function on a day-to-day basis
- Inexpensive and relatively easy test to perform

Microalbuminuria (MAU) Test for Kidney Function

Microalbumin is a protein that is normally absent from the urine or found in very small amounts when kidney function is normal. The purpose of the MAU test is to detect early microalbuminuria so that further decline in kidney function can be prevented or delayed.

The most commonly used test for albuminuria is the random spot urine sample to evaluate microalbumin-to-creatinine ratio. Results are interpreted as follows:
- Normal is less than 30 mcg/mg.
- Microalbuminuria is defined as 30 – 299 mcg/mg.
- Clinical albuminuria is ≥ 300 mcg/mg.

Repeat MAU testing is usually required to confirm findings, as several factors can influence the results. These factors include exercise within 24 hours of the test, infection, fever, inflammatory processes, hyperglycemia and hypertension. It is recommend that at least two of three tests performed within a 6-month period be elevated before confirming that the patient has microalbuminuria.

When clinical albuminuria is present, further testing of glomerular filtration rate (GFR) is indicated.

Liver Function Tests

Although diabetes is not known to directly affect liver function, most people with diabetes undergo routine liver function testing. Because polypharmacy is part of standard diabetes treatment, liver function tests are necessary to evaluate the safety of initiating medications and to monitor the effects of ongoing medication therapy on renal function.

Use of multiple medications increases the risk for drug interactions that cause inadequate clearance of byproducts from the liver. Elderly patients and patients who abuse alcohol are especially prone to impaired liver function. Caution should be used when prescribing medications that are metabolized by the liver.

The alanine aminotransferase (ALT) is a common liver function test for medication hepatotoxicity. The reference range for this test is 8 – 20 U/L.

Diabetes Burnout

Diabetes burnout results from the frustration of dealing with diabetes on a daily basis and leads to feelings of inadequacy and emotional depletion. Poor self-care practice is a symptom of diabetes burnout.

Ways the diabetes educator can help a client deal with diabetes burnout include:
- Acknowledging that living with diabetes is challenging and that many people with the disease have feelings of burnout.
- Developing a supportive and collaborative relationship with the client.
- Helping the client identify areas where he or she has been successful, as opposed to only pointing out shortcomings.
- Helping the client set reasonable, attainable goals.
- Encouraging the client to seek help and support from others and to optimize available resources.
- Helping the client develop effective problem-solving skills.

Adverse Affect on Social Relationships

Sometimes a support person becomes overly involved in a client's diabetes self-management. The support person might try to dictate and monitor what the person with diabetes should be doing without regard for the rights of the individual. This can be disempowering for the person with diabetes and can lead to power struggles in the relationship.

It is important to remember that the person with diabetes is the one with the rights and responsibilities related to his or her own diabetes care. The empowerment approach to self-care should be supported at every opportunity.

It is also important to recognize that a certain degree of dependency can be beneficial in a relationship. Therefore, the person with diabetes and the support person should openly discuss mutual expectations with regard to the management of diabetes. The feelings of the support person should be acknowledged, as they may include feelings of fear, grief and resentment. Referral to a mental health specialist is recommended when unhealthy behaviors are noted in a relationship.

Coping Skills

Assertiveness
- Being able to express feelings, wants and needs in a direct way
- Being able to say "no"
- Asking for help and clarification when needed

Positive self-talk
- Using positive language and speaking in terms that indicate optimism and hope
- Using language to support self-confidence, such as "I can do it"

Problem-solving
- Able to identify a problem
- Able to brainstorm possible solutions
- Able to select one or more realistic options for solving the problem

Priority setting and time management
- Able to differentiate between higher and lower priorities
- Able to organize and manage multiple priorities

Use of support system
- Can identify sources of help and support
- Able to specify how others can provide support

Diabetes and Depression

The rate of depression in people with diabetes is approximately three times that of people without diabetes. This condition affects about 15 – 20% of patients with diabetes. The causal relationship between the two conditions is unclear. It is not fully understood how one condition may cause the other or if there is bidirectional causation.

Depression has a negative impact on diabetes self-management. Studies show that depression is directly related to poor glycemic control and subsequent complications. This may be partly due to the association of depression with obesity, sedentary lifestyle and poor adherence to treatment recommendations. Diabetes complications shown to have a direct association with depression include retinopathy, neuropathic symptoms, nephropathy, hypertension and sexual dysfunction.

Depression is also associated with maladaptive coping methods, such as abuse of tobacco and other substances. This further increases the risk for cardiovascular disease, a risk already high in people with diabetes.

Atypical Symptoms of Depression

Depression is known to have a negative impact on glycemic control and to decrease tolerance to the physical symptoms related to diabetes. It has also been shown that reports of neuropathic pain, gastrointestinal problems and symptoms of hyperglycemia and hypoglycemia are more common among depressed people with diabetes.

Atypical symptoms of depression in the person with diabetes may include:
- Symptoms of hypoglycemia or hyperglycemia despite objective findings of glycemic control
- Physical symptoms that are out of proportion with objective data
- Sexual dysfunction
- Chronic pain
- Worsening of glycemic control
- Decline in self-care behavior
- Poor adaptation to diabetes

If these symptoms are identified, further evaluation for depression by standard means is required for diagnosis of the disorder.

Anxiety and Diabetes

It is common for clients to feel anxious about having diabetes. One study demonstrated that anxiety was elevated in 40% of subjects with diabetes. Anxiety is often experienced upon initial diagnosis of diabetes, at the onset of complications and during periods of poor glycemic control. People are often more receptive to outside help and support during these times, so they present an opportunity for providing education.

Diabetes-related anxieties often focus on the fear of hypoglycemia, complications, using insulin or performing fingersticks. Anxiety can also be manifested by compulsively checking blood glucose.

Depending upon the severity of the anxiety, emotional support, education and help with problem-solving can often alleviate anxiety related to diabetes. In other cases, referral to a mental health professional is warranted, especially if anxiety interferes with activities of daily living and effective self-care behavior.

Symptoms of Depression

Depression encompasses several mood disorders characterized by persistent feelings of sadness or lack of interest in usual activities.

Major Depressive Disorder (MDD) is the most common of these mood disorders. Diagnosis of MDD is based upon the presence of 5 out of 9 symptoms that the patient has experienced over a minimum of 2 weeks. These symptoms include sleep disturbance, unintended change in weight, difficulty in making decisions, fatigue, feelings of guilt or worthlessness and suicidal thoughts or plans.

Dysthymic Disorder is a disorder of prolonged depressive symptoms and results in greater impairment of social and vocational functioning.

Adjustment Disorder with Depressed Mood is depression that occurs within 3 months of an identified stressor, such as a death or job loss. This is a shorter-term condition and usually lasts 6 months or less.

Symptoms of Anxiety and Hypoglycemia

Anxiety disorders are common in adults in general and even more common in people with diabetes.

Common manifestations of anxiety include:
- Sleep disturbance
- Restlessness
- Muscle tension
- Agitation
- Irritability
- Lack of concentration
- Nervousness
- Poor memory
- Inability to make decisions

Clients with diabetes may exhibit anxiety by demonstrating irrational fears and refusing to perform certain aspects of self-care, such as monitoring blood glucose or injecting insulin.

Some of the symptoms of anxiety are similar to the symptoms of hypoglycemia. Clients who experience any symptoms of hypoglycemia should be instructed to check blood glucose when these symptoms appear. If the symptoms occur in spite of normal blood glucose, anxiety should be suspected as the cause.

Adherence in the Adolescent Client

Adherence to diabetes therapy is a challenge for any group, but probably more so for the adolescent. Some of the developmental issues of adolescence that impact treatment adherence include increased awareness of body image and differentiation from adult authority figures.

Strategies to help improve treatment adherence in the adolescent with type 1 diabetes include:
- Focus on what is relevant to the individual. For adolescents, this includes body image and peer relationships.
- Work with the client in establishing his or her own goals and be willing to compromise.
- Establish the primary relationship with the teen, but keep parents involved. Parental involvement is essential in prevention of ketoacidosis.
- Enhance feelings of normalcy.
- Involve the teen in peer support groups and diabetes camp.
- Maintain open lines of communication and explore perceived barriers.
- Provide positive reinforcement.

Beneficial Coping Skills

Reframing is a cognitive technique that can be an appropriate coping skill for people with diabetes. Using this technique, clients learn to identify thoughts and attitudes that trigger maladaptive behavior in challenging situations. Once the self-sabotaging thoughts are identified, the person can learn to restructure thoughts, feelings and attitudes in a more positive and productive way.

Relaxation techniques can also be effective in coping with the demands of diabetes. These may include progressive muscle relaxation, deep breathing and guided imagery.

Problem-solving skills are essential in coping with diabetes. Studies indicate that training in problem-solving improves glycemic control.

The effective use of a support system is another appropriate coping skill. Educators can help clients identify sources of support and guide them in specifying what they need from those around them.

Relapse prevention, another coping skill, may include maintaining an environment that supports a healthy lifestyle and having a system of rewards for staying on track.

Diabetes Self-Management

Role of the Client
The empowerment approach to diabetes management upholds that the person with diabetes has the rights and responsibilities for his or her care and management. This includes making the decision about when and how the individual will initiate and maintain self-care behaviors.

In adherence with this philosophy, the client's role includes:
- Identifying goals and setting an agenda for education
- Utilizing knowledge gained from education to make informed healthcare decisions
- Taking an active role in identifying problems and learning to problem-solve
- Participating in contracts with educators and other healthcare providers
- Identifying a support system and specifying the help needed

It is important to realize that clients have differing levels of comfort with self-care and some may prefer a more passive role. In these cases, it is best to support an incremental approach to developing self-management skills.

Role of the Educator
The empowerment approach advocates that the person with diabetes holds the rights and responsibilities for diabetes self-management. This differs from the compliance model in which the healthcare professional is perceived as the person having ultimate authority and responsibility.

In adherence with the empowerment approach, the roles of the educator include:
- Assisting clients to make informed decisions about their care and self-management
- Approaching education from the client's perspective and offering information relevant to the individual
- Identifying clients' readiness to change and providing stage-appropriate interventions
- Assisting clients to identify problems and helping them develop problem-solving skills
- Helping clients identify thoughts, feelings and attitudes that have an effect on diabetes self-management
- Assist with goal setting

Collaborative Relationship with Client

The empowerment approach to diabetes self-management education is built upon a foundation of collaboration between educator and client. In a collaborative relationship, the educator provides expertise and relevant information for safe decision-making on the part of the client. The client chooses how to use the information.

An important aspect of a collaborative client-educator relationship includes jointly setting and agreeing on an agenda. The agenda should start with things that are important to the client but should also include items the educator feels are important.

Working together to identify and solve problems is an important part of the collaborative relationship. The educator should resist the temptation to solve problems for the client, instead helping him or her identify possible solutions from which to choose.

A collaborative relationship relies upon active listening from the educator. This includes asking open-ended questions so that the client can verbalize thoughts, feelings and attitudes. Reflection and summarizing are also active listening techniques.

Role of the Family

Family support is an important component of successful diabetes self-management. Two important things to consider when involving the family in education are the cultural context of the family and the functional health and stability of family dynamics.

One role of the family is to learn about diabetes self-management along with the client. Ideally, this should begin at diagnosis and be maintained throughout the continuum of care. The educator can facilitate this by inviting family members to attend educational sessions with the client.

Family members' feelings about diabetes should be explored. These may include negative feelings based on erroneous information. The educator should help the family understand what is expected with regard to the client's blood glucose and behavior, so that their expectations will be realistic.

The family's role is to support the client. This may include supporting healthy eating as a family, engaging in physical activity together and working mutually to solve problems as they arise.

Variables in Decision to Make Behavioral Change

The transtheoretical model describes stages of psychological readiness that a person goes through in the behavior change process. This model stipulates that there are two major variables that affect the decision to make change.
- Decisional balance involves weighing the pros and cons of making the change. If the person perceives that the benefits and rewards of a behavior outweigh the costs and disadvantages, he or she is more likely to make the change.
- Self-efficacy is the person's self-confidence that he or she can actually initiate and maintain the proposed behavior change. The higher the self-efficacy, the greater the chance the person will make the change. Studies have indicated that self-efficacy is an important variable in diabetes self-management behaviors.

Motivational Interviewing

Motivational interviewing is a validated behavioral intervention technique that helps clients to explore ambivalence about change and to engage them in talking about change. It is usually most appropriate in one-to-one sessions.

Motivational interviewing elicits "change talk" from the client. The interviewer mirrors ambivalent statements made by the client and asks the client to reinforce the perceived benefits. Thus, by vocalizing one's own reasons for considering change, the client motivates him or herself to move toward change.

Another premise of motivational interviewing is to "roll with resistance." When a client is reluctant to engage in the recommended behavior, the interviewer explores the reasons for this rather than directly confronting the client.

Example of motivational interviewing: "It sounds like you have some reasons why you don't want to check your blood sugar regularly, yet you've indicated that you should be doing it more. What benefits do you think you would have by checking more often?"

Driver Safety

Patients who use sulfonylurea medications and insulin are at risk for hypoglycemia and should receive driver safety information. Non-sulfonylurea secretagogues, such as repaglinide, have a lower potential for causing hypoglycemia. Insulin poses the greatest risk.

Hypoglycemia can interfere with vision and mental processing, placing the person at high risk for accidents and injury. People at risk should wear medical identification to avoid being mistaken as driving while intoxicated.

Clients at risk should keep a fast-acting carbohydrate within arm's reach while driving. Good choices for the car include glucose tablets or a disposable juice box or bag.

Studies have indicated that many people underestimate the danger of driving with low blood glucose. Therefore, the educator should ask the client what he or she feels is a safe cutoff point.

The client should be instructed to test blood glucose prior to driving and to not drive if it is below 70 mg/dl.

Dental Issues

People with diabetes have a three-fold risk for such dental problems as caries, periodontal disease and tooth loss. Studies have indicated that people with diabetes underestimate the importance of good dental care and do not appreciate the relationship of good oral health with general health.

Dental problems can negatively affect glycemic control, while poor glycemic control can complicate dental visits and procedures. Common issues related to diabetes that complicate dental care include poor wound healing, susceptibility for infection, vascular changes and neuropathy.

Tooth loss or dental pain can affect what a person is able to eat and can lead to insufficient intake of healthy foods such as vegetables, fruits and whole grains. Softer foods tend to cause a sharper rise in blood glucose.

Dental treatments, such as root canals or oral surgery, can require changes in food intake and adjustment in oral medications and insulin.

Promoting Good Dental Health
Educators should consider teaching about dental care as a standard component of the diabetes education program. The following points should be included:

- There is an interrelationship between dental health and glycemic control. A decline in one can lead to a decline in the other.
- Maintain glycemic control and healthy eating habits.
- Maintain good routine brushing and flossing habits.
- See the dentist every 6 months—more often if there is periodontal disease.
- Notify the dentist that you have diabetes and know your most recent A1C value.
- Don't smoke, as it increases the risk for periodontal disease.
- Dry mouth, common in diabetes, promotes the formation of dental caries. Maintain good hydration and use fluoride mouth rinses and salivary substitutes as needed.
- Be prepared to make adjustments in food, oral medication and insulin for dental procedures.

Interventions for Periodontal Disease
People with diabetes have a higher risk for periodontal disease; the risk is even greater in those who smoke. Increased age and longer duration of diabetes are also risk factors for periodontal disease.

Periodontal disease should be suspected with the following presentation:

- History of poor glycemic control
- Current and persistent poor glycemic control with no obvious reason
- Red, inflamed, tender gums
- Bleeding gums
- Foul breath odor
- Change in eating habits to soft foods

When periodontal disease is suspected, interventions include:

- Educating the client that gum disease can negatively affect control of blood glucose
- Referring to a dental health professional
- Continuing to work with the client to lower blood glucose levels
- Anticipating dietary changes, such as consuming more soft foods, that can have an influence on blood glucose control

Dental Visit Safety Factors
People with diabetes have a greater risk for dental caries, periodontal disease and other dental problems. Poor glycemic control is associated with impaired wound healing and increased susceptibility for infection. Dental procedures with sedation may require fasting prior to the procedure while post-procedural pain may affect what the person is able to eat afterward.

Teaching points for safety related to dental care and procedures includes:

- Notify your dentist that you have diabetes and know your most recent A1C result.
- Prevent hypoglycemia during examinations and procedures by having appropriate food intake before the dental visit.
- If fasting is required before a procedure, be aware that a reduction in medication or insulin may be necessary.
- Avoid scheduling a dental appointment during the hours when insulin action will be peaking.

- If at risk for hypoglycemia, have at least 15 grams of fasting-acting carbohydrate readily available.
- Avoid dental surgeries during periods of severe hyperglycemia, as this will affect healing and increase the risk for infection.

Skin Problems

- Anhidrosis – An autonomic neuropathic condition which leads to little or no production of perspiration in the feet and lower legs, resulting in severely dry and cracked skin.
- Diabetic dermopathy – Pigmented spots on the shins, usually asymptomatic but can be painful if they ulcerate. Most likely due to poor skin perfusion associated with diabetes.
- Acanthosis nigricans – Velvety brown or black lesions found in the folds of the skin, most commonly the folds of the neck and axillae. The condition is associated with obesity and insulin resistance. In the young, it is a marker of glucose intolerance and when present should prompt providers to screen for type 2 diabetes.
- Skin infections – High risk for skin infections is associated with poor glycemic control, as well as neuropathy and peripheral vascular disease. Common skin infections in diabetes include staph, fungal and Candida infections.

Skin Care

Elevated glucose can cause dry skin and increase the risk for skin infections. Common skin infections in people with diabetes include staph, beta-hemolytic strep, fungal, and yeast infections. Furthermore, comorbidities such as neuropathy and peripheral vascular disease can complicate infections and slow healing.

Teaching points for skin care include:
- Maintain glycemic control.
- Maintain healthy eating habits and adequate hydration status.
- Inspect skin daily and report infections promptly to a healthcare provider.
- Pay attention to skinfold areas where fungus and yeast tend to grow. Dry well in all skinfolds, including between the toes, after each bath or shower. Antifungal powders may be used in skinfolds and shoes.
- Avoid trauma to the skin.
- Wear protective footwear.
- Avoid overexposure to the sun, especially if taking sulfonylurea medication.
- Use mild soap to bathe and avoid harsh or drying skin care products, such as those that contain alcohol.

Foot Care

Education about foot care should be individualized to the client's current level of knowledge, risk level and foot care practices. Foot care practices should be discussed with high-risk clients at every visit.

The educator should begin by asking what the client already knows about foot care and what he or she is currently doing for foot care. Open-ended questions are best.

Special situations that may alter one's ability to perform good foot care may include homelessness, blindness and obesity.

Instruction should be presented in a positive way with rationales.

Carefully selected handouts and written guidelines can be helpful. Handouts should be screened for literacy level and cultural appropriateness. Graphic presentations are often desirable. Handouts should be provided in the client's preferred language.

<u>Self-Foot Exam</u>
Patients with neuropathy and loss of protective sensation should perform a self-foot exam every day. While those who maintain good sensation are at lower risk for serious foot problems, checking the feet every day is a good practice for all people with diabetes.

To check the feet, instruct the client to:
- Carefully inspect all surfaces of the feet, including top, bottom and between toes.
- Note any areas of skin breakdown or irritation. Report infection or slow healing to a healthcare provider promptly.
- Note areas that indicate poorly fitting shoes, such as callus formation or red pressure areas upon removing shoes.
- Use a mirror if needed to visually access all areas of the feet. Enlist the help of a support person if necessary.

It is helpful to have the client provide a return demonstration of the foot inspection instruction that has been given.

<u>Teaching Points for Foot Care</u>
Inspect feet daily.

Inspect shoes for irregularities that may cause pressure or irritate skin. Shake out shoes before putting them on.

Always wear well-fitting, protective shoes and socks.

Wash feet daily with mild soap and warm water as part of the bath or shower. Foot soaks are not recommended. Dry the feet after the bath or shower, especially between the toes.

Use moisturizer for dry skin. Avoid getting it between the toes. Avoid highly scented moisturizers and those containing alcohol, which may irritate or dry the skin.

For calluses, gently rub with a pumice stone after the bath or shower, followed by application of moisturizing cream or lotion. Do not use sharp instruments to cut a callus and do not use over-the-counter treatments containing harsh chemicals that may burn the skin.

Cut toenails straight across.

Do not use heating pads or hot water bottles to warm the feet.

Promptly report any problems, such as cuts, scrapes or blisters that do not heal or appear to be infected.

Economic Burden of Diabetes

Diabetes exacts a heavy economic burden upon the individual and society, with healthcare expenditures for people with the disease averaging 2 – 3 times that of the general population. In addition, many of those with diabetes have decreased earning potential due to disability imposed by the disease.

The Social Security Disability Insurance (SSDI) program provides assistance to disabled workers and their families. The government reported that there were 122,000 cases in which diabetes was the primary basis for disability in 2002.

Costs to the individual are high and include insurance premiums, co-pays, multiple prescription medications, testing supplies and durable medical equipment. Studies show that many people do not take all of their prescribed medication due to the cost.

Socioeconomic Status and Utilization of Dental Care

Because diabetes increases the risk for dental problems and because dental problems can affect glycemic control, regular dental care is an important part of diabetes management.

There is a strong relationship between socioeconomic status and utilization of dental services. Dental care is often not covered by insurance to the same extent that medical insurance covers health care, so it represents a much greater out-of-pocket expense to patients. Furthermore, Medicare does not provide for dental care and Medicaid provides only limited coverage for dental care in some states.

A recent study has shown that, among people with diabetes, there is a greater disparity in utilization of professional dental care based upon racial, ethnic and socioeconomic status than for any other type of health care. Those with an income of less than $10,000 saw a dentist at roughly half the rate of those with income over $50,000. These disparities did not exist for physician visits or foot exams among the same groups.

Self-Monitoring of Blood Glucose

Select and Prepare the Fingertip

Capillary blood, usually from the fingertip, is used for self-monitoring of blood glucose (SMBG). Fingertip testing is more comfortable when the prick is situated along the sides of the fingertip, rather than the tip or the pad where more nerve endings are clustered. The client should also select a site that does not have callus formation and rotate testing sites.

Inadequate blood sample is one of the most common user errors in SMBG. Tips for helping a client get an adequate sample from the fingertip include:
- Wash hands vigorously with warm water prior to testing.
- Dangle hand below the waist and shake it for 30 – 60 seconds to increase blood flow.
- Gently milk the finger after the puncture rather than squeeze it.
- Adjust the depth of puncture on the lancing device if necessary.

<u>Alternate Sites (Other Than The Fingertip) For Collecting A Blood Sample</u>
Obtaining capillary blood from the fingertip is the most common method for self-monitoring of blood glucose (SMBG). Some clients prefer alternate-site testing to avoid repeated pricks to the sensitive areas of the fingertips. Alternate sites include the fleshy parts of the palm of the hand, such as the thenar aspect, as well as the forearm, abdomen or thigh. Clients should only perform alternate-site testing if approved by the manufacturer of their equipment and the proper device for pricking is used. Often a special end cap to the lancing device is required.

Obtaining a blood drop from alternate sites can be more challenging than getting blood from the fingertip. It takes more time for the blood drop to form from these other sites. The lancing device usually needs to be held firmly on the site for several seconds before and after the puncture to produce the drop. Gently rubbing the site for 30 – 60 seconds before testing may improve blood flow. Instruct the client to follow the manufacturer's instructions for how to place and hold the lancing device on the site.

Continuous Glucose Monitoring

Continuous glucose monitoring (CGM) is a newer technology that is gaining more widespread use. The device uses a sensor to measure the glucose of interstitial tissue on a continuous basis. This type of monitoring is most appropriate for those on intensive insulin regimens as the close, real-time monitoring allows for on-the-spot insulin adjustments. Because there is a 2 – 3 minute lag between interstitial glucose and capillary blood glucose, alarms for hypoglycemia should be set to go off at a higher-than-usual target to allow for prompt detection of hypoglycemia.

Careful client selection for CGM is important. Insurance reimbursement for CGM is minimal, so many clients cannot afford the device. Clients selected for CGM should have the cognitive skills and desire to work with technology and be able to use a software system to analyze blood glucose data.

Selecting a Blood Glucose Meter

The insurance formulary often dictates the choices available to the client. In general, all meters meet similar criteria for accuracy as long as the manufacturer's instructions are followed. Test strips for the various meters are comparatively priced.

A plasma-referenced meter may be preferred over a meter that reports results as whole blood. While all meters use a whole blood sample, laboratory glucose values are reported from plasma. Meters that self-calibrate to report results as a plasma value allow better comparison between home and laboratory results.

Some clients may need a meter that helps them adapt to functional limitations in vision, manual dexterity or cognition. Some meters have strips that come in a cassette that helps reduce the need for inserting a strip into the meter each time. Other meters require fewer steps in the procedure and some have larger screens.

Some clients' lifestyles, occupations or preferences may indicate that a meter allowing for alternate-site testing is the best choice.

Clients who like technology may prefer a meter with advanced electronic features and data management capabilities.

Ketone Testing

Ketones, which are byproducts of fat metabolism, can cause acidosis when present in excessive amounts. People with type 1 diabetes are prone to ketosis while those with type 2 diabetes are usually ketone-resistant.

People with type 2 diabetes are most likely to experience ketosis during periods of acute illness or following trauma. Therefore, they should test for ketones during these times.

People with type 1 diabetes should monitor ketones whenever their blood glucose is consistently > 300 mg/dl and when ill.

Measuring ketones may also be considered in all patients with diabetes who are trying to lose weight by calorie restriction.

Ketones can be measured in the blood or urine. Special meters for home use are available for measuring blood ketones while dipsticks are used for the urine.

Estimated Average Glucose

The A1C test is the gold standard for monitoring blood glucose control. By measuring the degree of glycation of the red blood cells, it provides a picture of blood glucose control over the previous 2 – 3 months. There is a linear relationship between A1C and blood glucose, so as one goes up or down, so does the other.

Recent research has refined a formula for correlating blood glucose and A1C values (see table below for the correlations). This is called estimated average glucose (eAG). Its purpose is to help patients better interpret their A1C in relation to their self-monitoring.

The American Diabetes Association advocates using the eAG to enhance communication with patients about the results of their laboratory values. Using mg/dl as the unit of measure for reporting results is thought to be more understandable to patients, as this is what they are accustomed to seeing on their home testing equipment.

6%	126 mg/dl
6.5%	140 mg/dl
7%	154 mg/dl
7.5%	169 mg/dl
8%	183 mg/dl

Metabolic Monitoring to Prevent Cardiovascular Disease

Because cardiovascular disease is the leading cause of death among people with diabetes, measures to prevent heart attack and stroke in these patients are paramount. Studies show that reducing risk factors saves lives.

While monitoring blood pressure and lipids are essential to risk management, it should be noted that microalbuminuria is another important marker of cardiovascular risk.

Blood pressure should be monitored at every visit. The target blood pressure goal for people with diabetes is 130/80 mmHg.

Fasting lipid levels should be measured at least annually. Target goals, according to the American Diabetes Association are:
- LDL-C < 100 mg/dl
- HDL-C > 40 mg/dl (men)
- HDL-C > 50 mg/dl (women)
- Triglycerides < 150 mg/dl

Urine microalbumin should be measured annually, starting at 5 years after diagnosis in type 1 diabetes and upon diagnosis in type 2 diabetes. The normal value for spot urine collection is < 30 mcg/mg.

Pattern Management

Normally, pattern management involves observing and recording blood glucose for 2 – 3 days and making insulin adjustments based upon a pattern of high or low blood glucose at a given time of day. However, for very high blood glucose values, supplemental insulin can be taken immediately.

Changes in insulin doses are made according to the time of day being observed and the type of insulin being used. Although treatment regimens are always individualized, a rule of thumb is to adjust only after a pattern is observed for 2 – 3 days and changes are made in 10 – 20% increments until target blood glucose is achieved.

Examples of insulin adjustments in response to patterns include:
- Glucose high or low before breakfast → Adjust bedtime intermediate (NPH) or long-acting (glargine, detemir) insulin
- Glucose high after breakfast → Adjust pre-breakfast rapid-acting insulin
- Glucose high after lunch → Adjust pre-lunch rapid-acting insulin
- Glucose high after dinner → Adjust pre-dinner rapid-acting insulin

Handwritten vs. Downloaded Blood Glucose Records

Handwritten records offer greater opportunity to keep a journal of factors that affect blood glucose and may provide more opportunity for problem-solving than downloaded records. With written records, the person with diabetes may be able to more clearly associate such things as food, activity, stress, emotions and medications to blood glucose results.

Cables and software for downloading meter results are available from most meter manufacturers. Downloading blood glucose records may be more convenient for some people and make testing and recordkeeping more portable. Many providers prefer downloaded records from their patients. When patients use downloaded records exclusively, they may miss opportunities to make important adjustments to the meal or exercise plans or the medication regimen.

Medical Nutrition Therapy

The nutrition recommendations and interventions for diabetes are published by the American Diabetes Association (ADA) to provide science-based evidence to people with diabetes and their healthcare providers. Medical nutrition therapy (MNT) is appropriate at all levels along the diabetes care continuum, from primary prevention of diabetes to prevention and management of complications and prevention of morbidity and mortality.

The ADA recommendations stipulate that the person with diabetes is central to the nutritional management team and plays an active role in decision-making. While supporting the goals of MNT is considered a team effort, it is recommended that a registered dietitian play the leading role. At the same time, other healthcare providers, such as doctors and nurses, should be knowledgeable about these guidelines and play and active role in their implementation.

Goals of Medical Nutrition Therapy
Medical nutrition therapy (MNT) is an integral part of diabetes management throughout the continuum of care.

According to the American Diabetes Association, the goals of MNT for diabetes are to:
- Achieve and maintain glycemic control
- Achieve and maintain a lipid profile that will reduce the risk for cardiovascular disease
- Achieve and maintain blood pressure at target level
- Prevent or delay long-term complications of diabetes
- Individualize nutritional needs based on personal and cultural preferences and willingness to change eating habits
- Integrate the meal plan with the insulin regimen if the patient uses insulin
- Maintain eating as a pleasurable activity with limitations based on scientific evidence
- Meet the concurrent nutritional needs of people with diabetes at different times in the lifecycle, such as youth, pregnancy, lactation and old age
- Safely coordinate nutritional recommendations with risk for hypoglycemia.

Nutrition Recommendations for Prevention of Diabetes

The Diabetes Prevention Program and other studies have demonstrated that type 2 diabetes can be prevented in high-risk, overweight people through intensive lifestyle modification.

Nutrition recommendations and interventions for the prevention of type 2 diabetes include:
- Moderate weight loss of 7% of body weight
- 150 minutes of moderate physical activity per week
- Dietary reduction of fat and calories
- Dietary fiber intake of 14 gram/1,000 kcal, with one-half of grain intake coming from whole grains

There are no nutritional recommendations for the prevention of type 1 diabetes.

Data for preventing diabetes in youth is unavailable. However the ADA proposes that the same measures demonstrated to be effective in adults would be appropriate for children as long as growth and developmental needs are met.

Micronutrient Requirements for Diabetes

Evidence does not support specific vitamin or mineral supplements to benefit people with diabetes. Getting adequate micronutrients from natural foods and a healthy, well-balanced diet is encouraged. Multivitamin supplementation may be appropriate in elderly clients, strict vegetarians and those on calorie-restricted diets, as well as in pregnant and lactating women.

The American Diabetes Association (ADA) states that further research is needed on such micronutrients as chromium and magnesium before they would be recommended for diabetes management.

The benefit of antioxidant supplementation in people with diabetes has been studied since diabetes is a state of increased oxidative stress. So far, there is no evidence that antioxidant therapy improves glycemic control or reduces the risk for long-term complications. In fact, there is evidence that that supplementation with vitamin E, carotene and other antioxidants is potentially harmful.

General Nutritional Recommendations for Diabetes

There is not a single "diabetic diet." Medical nutrition therapy (MNT) is a process provided by a registered dietitian to assess and diagnose a client's nutritional status and to make individualized dietary recommendations.

The general principles of the meal plan for diabetes include:
- If overweight, start by losing 5 – 7% of body weight. Even modest weight loss can produce significant results in glucose and lipid results. For overweight clients, achieving weight loss shares priority status with achieving glycemic control.
- Eat consistent amounts of carbohydrates from day to day and distribute evenly throughout the day. While eating sugar is not forbidden, the daily intake of carbohydrate should be monitored and controlled.
- Practice portion control.
- Limit fats in the diet, especially saturated fats and trans fats.
- Engage in 150 minutes of moderate intensity physical activity every week.

Utilize blood glucose monitoring results to evaluate the effect of food type, portion size, timing of meals and physical activity on blood glucose level.

Daily Calories, Macronutrients, Sodium And Fiber
Calories – 11 kcal/pound of ideal body weight for weight maintenance (more for those who are more physically active and less for weight loss).

Carbohydrates – 130 gram/day minimum; should comprise 45 – 65% of total calories.
Protein – Should make up about 15 – 20% of daily caloric intake; there are 7 grams of protein per ounce.

Fat – Total intake is individualized, but usually recommended to be 25 – 30% of daily calories. Less than 7% of calories should come from saturated fat. For individual foods, the goal is to have <1 gram of saturated fat per 100 calories. Daily intake of trans fats should be zero.

Sodium – Moderate sodium intake is considered 2,300 – 2,400 mg/day. For hypertension, reduction to 1,500 mg/day is recommended. One teaspoon of salt contains 2,300 mg of sodium.

Fiber – At least 14 grams of fiber per 1,000 calories. Some studies show greater amounts have a beneficial effect on glycemic control.

ADA Recommendations for Carbohydrate in Nutritional Management of Diabetes
Dietary carbohydrate is the major determinant of postprandial blood glucose excursions. While carbohydrate limitation is beneficial, carbohydrates cannot be eliminated from the diet as they are an important source of fiber, vitamins and minerals.

Below is a summary of the ADA nutrition recommendations for carbohydrate in diabetes management:
- A balanced diet including carbohydrate from fruit, vegetables, whole grains, legumes and low-fat milk is encouraged.
- People with diabetes should monitor carbohydrate intake by a method such as carbohydrate counting, food exchanges or visual estimation.
- Use of the glycemic index may be an appropriate supplement to monitoring total carbohydrate intake.
- Sugar, such as sucrose, can be substituted for other carbohydrate in the meal plan. If sugar is added, additional insulin or exercise may be indicated.
- Although a specific value for fiber intake has not been determined for people with diabetes, a diet rich in fiber is recommended.
- Non-nutritive sugar substitutes and sugar alcohols are safe when used within guidelines established by the Food and Drug Administration.

Implications of Sodium in Medical Nutrition Therapy
As part of the metabolic syndrome, hypertension is a common finding in clients with diabetes. People with diabetes also tend to be more salt-sensitive than the general population, meaning that reductions in sodium intake are more likely to have a beneficial effect on blood pressure. As a population, African Americans tend to have a high degree of sodium sensitivity.

Moderate sodium intake is considered 2,300 – 2,400 mg/day. For hypertension a reduction to 1,500 mg/ day is often recommended.

Clients should be instructed to look for the sodium content of foods on food labels. It is listed as mg of sodium per serving. For single-serving foods, 400 mg or less of sodium is recommended. For an entrée, less than 800 mg of sodium is recommended. A food labeled "low sodium" has 140 mg or less of sodium per serving.

A teaspoon of salt contains 2,300 mg of sodium.

Glycemic Index in Nutritional Management

Many factors influence the postprandial glucose response to carbohydrate ingestion. These factors include the type of starch (amylase versus amylopectin), degree of processing, the composition of the meal, method of cooking, the ripeness of the plant and the insulin availability or sensitivity of the individual.

The glycemic index compares the postprandial response of carbohydrate-containing foods. The glycemic response of a food is compared to the glucose response of a reference food, such as white bread or rice. The glycemic index is the rise in blood glucose at 2 hours following ingestion of a 50-gram carbohydrate portion.

Low glycemic index foods include oats, legumes, pumpernickel bread, apples and oranges.

Research results are conflicting on the efficacy of the glycemic index in diabetes management and methodological problems exist. How a food is processed or where it is grown can cause variability in the glycemic index of the same type of food. The ripeness of a fruit or vegetable can also account for variability among the same foods.

Fiber Intake for People with Diabetes

While there is not a specific recommendation for fiber intake in the management of diabetes, a diet high in fiber is encouraged. People with diabetes are encouraged to at least strive for a dietary intake of fiber that matches the USDA recommendation for the general population, which is 14 grams/1,000 kcal. Research indicates that a high-fiber diet (approximately 50 grams of fiber per day) is associated with reduced glycemia in people with type 1 diabetes and reduced glycemia and lipemia in people with type 2 diabetes.

Foods containing ≥ 5 grams/serving are considered rich in fiber and should be encouraged. Examples include legumes, fiber-rich cereals and many whole grain products. Barriers to adhering to a high-fiber diet include gastrointestinal side effects, palatability and limited food choices.

Carbohydrate Counting

In carbohydrate counting, the client adds the total amount of carbohydrate being consumed. Done properly, it can provide a healthy, balanced diet with controlled portions of carbohydrate.

One carbohydrate serving equals 15 grams of carbohydrate. The client selects the correct number of carbohydrate servings to meet their recommended allowance.

Examples of 15-gram carbohydrate servings include:
- 1 small piece of fruit
- $\frac{1}{3}$ cup rice, cooked
- $\frac{1}{3}$ cup pasta, cooked
- 1 cup milk
- $\frac{3}{4}$ cup yogurt
- 1 slice bread
- 1 small potato

Nonstarchy vegetables contain approximately 5 grams of carbohydrate per cup. If eaten in moderate amounts, they are usually not counted in the allowance. If a large amount is eaten, nonstarchy vegetables should be counted.

"Free foods," which contain less than 20 calories and fewer than 5 grams of carbohydrate per serving, are not counted. These include pickles, salsa, many condiments and sugar-free gelatin.

Typical Meal Plan for Type 2 Diabetes, Using the Carbohydrate Counting Method
For carbohydrate counting, the client is given an allowance of how many carbohydrate choices are allowed for each meal and snack.

A typical carbohydrate counting meal plan allows 3 to 4 carbohydrate choices per meal. Each carbohydrate choice, or serving, equals 15 grams. Examples of serving sizes are 1 small piece of fruit, 1 slice of bread or $\frac{1}{3}$ cup of cooked rice. Some clients also receive an additional allowance of 1 – 2 carbohydrate choices for snacks each day.

Clients select, or mix and match the carbohydrates of their choice to equal the allowance for the meal. The type of carbohydrate is not specified, only the amount. Consistency of carbohydrate intake helps stabilize the blood glucose, no matter the source. Care should be taken to limit carbohydrate choices that are high in fat and calories.

The carbohydrate allowance recommendation is based upon factors such as gender, physical activity level and medications. Blood glucose logs help in evaluating results and optimizing the recommendation.

Sucrose and Fructose

There is strong evidence that, in equal caloric amounts, dietary sucrose does not increase blood glucose more than starch. Therefore, the intake of sugar and sweet foods is not forbidden to people with diabetes. Sucrose can be substituted for equivalent amounts of starch without a significant difference in effect on glycemia. However, clients should be cautioned to avoid excessive caloric intake of sweets and to possibly increase insulin or other glucose-lowering medication when sugar is added to the diet.

Fructose has a lower glycemic index than either sucrose or starch. However, adding fructose as a sweetening agent is not recommended because of its adverse effect on plasma lipids. Naturally occurring fructose in fruits and other foods does not need to be eliminated from the diet if these foods account for only 3 – 4% of total energy intake.

Sugar Alcohols and Non-Nutritive Sweeteners

Sugar alcohols are reduced-calorie sweeteners such as isomalt, maltilol, sorbitol, xylitol and hydrogenated starch hydrolysates. When ingested, these substances have reduced glycemic effect when compared to sucrose and glucose. They contain about half the calories of sucrose. Sugar alcohols are also associated with decreased risk for dental caries. Side effects of consuming sugar alcohols are abdominal discomfort and diarrhea. When counting the carbohydrates of a food containing sugar alcohols, it is appropriate to subtract half of the sugar alcohol grams from the total carbohydrates.

There are five non-nutritive sweeteners approved by the Food and Drug Administration. All have undergone rigorous testing and have been determined safe for human consumption, including people with diabetes and pregnant women. The approved non-nutritive sweeteners are acesulfame potassium, aspartame, neotame, saccharin and sucralose.

Dietary Fats

Saturated fats raise LDL-C levels. Less than 7% of daily calories should come from these. Sources include animal fat and coconut, palm and hydrogenated vegetable oils.

Trans fatty acids, a form of saturated fats, are found in processed foods, such as boxed dinners and baked goods. Their intake should be restricted.

Polyunsaturated fats lower total cholesterol but have a mixed effect on HDL-C levels. Sources are corn and sunflower oils and walnuts. Intake should be less than 10% of daily calories.

Monounsaturated fats lower total cholesterol but do not lower HDL-C. They are more beneficial to the lipid panel than polyunsaturated oils. Sources include nuts and canola, olive and peanut oils.

Omega-3 polyunsaturated fats lower serum triglycerides and have an antiplatelet clotting effect. Sources include fatty fish such as salmon, herring and sardines as well as flaxseed and walnuts.

Dietary cholesterol raises cholesterol levels in some people more than others. Intake should be less than 200 – 300 mg/day. Sources are egg yolks, organ meats and dairy fat.

ADA Recommendations for Dietary Fat and Cholesterol
Since cardiovascular risk is high in people with diabetes, a primary goal in their dietary management is to limit saturated fats, trans fatty acids and cholesterol. Saturated fats and trans fatty acids are the fats that affect the LDL-C level.

The effects of diets having specific percentages of saturated fats, trans fatty acids and cholesterol on people with diabetes have not been adequately studied. Therefore, recommendations are based on the guidelines for people with pre-existing cardiovascular disease, since the risk among the two groups is relatively equivalent.

The ADA recommendations for dietary fat and cholesterol management are:
- Saturated fat intake limited to < 7% of total caloric intake
- Minimal intake of food containing trans fat
- Dietary cholesterol intake < 200 mg/day
- Two or more servings of fish per week (excluding commercially fried fish filets)

Protein

Although 50 – 60% of ingested protein converts to glucose, it is not known for certain where this glucose goes. Researchers have suggested that it is probably stored in the liver or muscle as glycogen. In those with poor glycemic control, gluconeogenesis following protein consumption can happen rapidly and cause an increase in blood glucose. For those with type 2 diabetes in good control, protein consumption does not increase plasma glucose levels.

Contrary to popular belief, consuming protein simultaneously with carbohydrate does not slow the blood glucose response to carbohydrate or have an effect on its peak activity. Consuming protein following treatment of a hypoglycemic episode does not prevent recurrence of the hypoglycemia. Similarly, consuming protein at bedtime or prior to exercise has not proven beneficial in preventing nocturnal hypoglycemia. The current recommendation for insulin users is to reduce insulin dose or consume a snack, either carbohydrate alone or with protein, prior to bedtime.

ADA Recommendations for Dietary Protein

The recommended dietary intake of protein for people with diabetes is the similar to that for the general population and generally does not exceed 20% of daily energy intake. Examples of good-quality protein sources include meat, poultry, fish, eggs, milk, cheese and soy.

Although some studies indicate that a high-protein diet may have a positive effect on glycemic control and can reduce appetite, these diets are not recommended for people with diabetes, even those having normal kidney function, due to lack of adequate evidence regarding their safety and efficacy.

ADA recommendations for protein in the management of diabetes are summarized as follows:
- Protein intake should be similar to that of the general population in the person with diabetes having normal renal function.
- Protein is not effective in treating hypoglycemia and should not be used to prevent nighttime hypoglycemia since it can increase insulin response without increasing plasma glucose.
- High-protein diets are not recommended for weight loss, even in patients with normal renal function.

Protein Restriction for Chronic Kidney Disease

The progression of the microvascular complications of diabetes may be moderated by decreasing protein in the diet, along with attaining glycemic control and lowering blood pressure.

The usual dietary intake of protein for Americans is 1.2 – 1.4 g/kg of body weight per day, or approximately 15 – 20% of daily energy.

For microalbuminuria: Studies show that reducing protein to 0.8 – 1.0 g/kg of body weight per day has a beneficial effect on renal function.

For clinical nephropathy: Reducing the amount to 0.8 g/kg of body weight per day improves measures of renal function.

Reducing protein intake to less than 0.8 g/kg of body weight per day is controversial. Limitation of protein should not preclude maintaining adequate nutritional status of the patient with CKD.

Integrating Food and Insulin

For people using insulin and oral glucose-lowering medications, the treatment plan should integrate the medication with food intake and the physical activity pattern. The approach to this depends upon the individual's medication, preferred meal pattern and physical activity pattern.

For those on basal bolus insulin regimens, the individual will count carbohydrates and inject the corresponding amount of rapid-acting insulin prior to the meal according to the established insulin-to-carbohydrate ratio. This applies to clients on either an insulin pump or multiple daily injections.

For clients on fixed insulin doses and oral glucose-lowering medications, daily carbohydrate consumption should remain consistent.

For planned exercise, decreasing the insulin dosage is recommended to prevent hypoglycemia. For unplanned exercise, carbohydrate intake will need to be increased to prevent hypoglycemia. Clients taking oral insulin secretagogues may need to lower the daily dose when undertaking an ongoing and consistent pattern of increased physical activity.

Food Labels for Carbohydrate Counting

Clients who are carbohydrate counting should be taught to prioritize the information they find on the "Nutrition Facts" food label.

The first thing to determine is the serving size. All other values on the label are based upon the specified serving size.

Next, the client should look at the total carbohydrate value. This reports the combined number of carbohydrate grams from sugar, starch and fiber that corresponds with the serving size. Clients should compare this to the 15-gram carbohydrate serving used in the carbohydrate counting meal plan. Many clients need to be instructed to ignore the grams of sugar reported on the label, as this is already included in the total carbohydrate figure.

Lastly, clients should check the food label for fiber content. If a food has more than 5 grams of fiber per serving, they can subtract that amount from the total carbohydrate and use the difference when figuring their carbohydrate intake.

Descriptive Terms And Health Claims Used On Food Labels

Descriptions of food products, such as "fat-free" and "no sugar added," are regulated by law. In order for manufacturers to make such claims, a food must comply with its intended definition.

Examples of some descriptive terms and their meanings:
- Fat free – $\frac{1}{2}$ gram or less per serving
- Low fat – 3 grams or less per serving
- Reduced fat – At least 25% less fat than the regular version of a food
- Sugar free – $\frac{1}{2}$ gram or less per serving
- No sugar added – No sugar or fruit juice added during processing
- Reduced sugar – Less than 25% of the sugar in the regular version
- Light or lite – 50% less fat or $\frac{1}{3}$ fewer calories than the regular version

Certain health claims on food packaging must be approved by the Food and Drug Administration. Examples:
- If a food is high in fiber, the package can claim that it helps reduce risk for cancer and heart disease.
- The label for a food low in sodium can claim that it helps prevent hypertension.

ADA Guidelines for Alcohol

While some people with diabetes can safely drink alcohol in moderation, abstinence is advised for those who are pregnant, have a history of alcohol abuse or have liver disease, severely elevated triglycerides or other contraindicating medical conditions.

Moderation means drinking less than one alcoholic beverage per day for women and less than two a day for men. One serving of alcohol equals 12 oz beer, 5 oz wine or 1.5 oz distilled spirits.

When consumed with food, alcohol has minimal immediate effect on glycemia. When ingested with carbohydrate, it can raise the blood glucose. For those taking insulin or insulin secretagogues, alcohol can cause hypoglycemia.

ADA guidelines for alcohol use are summarized as follows:
- People with diabetes who choose to use alcohol should do so in moderation.
- Alcohol should be consumed with food to reduce the risk for nocturnal hypoglycemia in people using insulin and glucose-lowering oral agents.
- Drinks mixed with carbohydrate, such as juice or soda, should be avoided to prevent high blood glucose.

Weight Control

Overweight vs. Obesity
The body mass index (BMI) is a commonly used screening tool to identify weight problems and associated health risks. Calculated from a person's height and weight, it is highly correlated to obesity or fat mass and risk for disease. The BMI classifications according to the National Heart, Lung and Blood Institute are:
- Normal: 18.5 – 24.9
- Overweight, increased risk for disease: 25 – 29.9
- Obese, high risk: 30.0 – 34.9
- Very high risk: 35.0 – 39.9
- Extremely high risk: ≥ 40

Waist circumference is a measure of visceral body fat. This is useful because excessive abdominal fat is a risk factor for type 2 diabetes, hypertension, dyslipidemia and cardiovascular disease (CVD). Excess waist circumference with associated health risk is identified as:
- Men – > 40 inches
- Women (non-pregnant) – > 35 inches

ADA Recommendations for Weight Loss
There is strong evidence that moderate weight loss increases insulin sensitivity in overweight and obese people with insulin resistance. ADA recommendations for weight loss include:
- Moderate weight loss for overweight or obese people who have diabetes or who are at risk for diabetes.
- Weight loss can be achieved through either low-carbohydrate or low-fat, calorie-restricted diets followed for up to one year.
- Exercise and behavior modification are essential components of any weight loss plan.

- Weight loss medications may be appropriate for some overweight or obese people with diabetes if combined with lifestyle modification.
- Bariatric surgery may be appropriate for some obese people with diabetes and a BMI ≥ 35.

Lipid profiles and renal function should be monitored for those on low-carbohydrate diets. Protein intake should be monitored in patients with nephropathy who are on a low-carbohydrate diet. Low-carbohydrate diets should be adjusted for prevention and treatment of hypoglycemia.

Successful Weight Loss and Long–Term Weight Management
Scientific evidence demonstrates that certain factors are necessary for successful long-term weight management. Components of the most successful programs are:
- Structured and intensive lifestyle modification
- Participant education
- Individualized counseling
- Calorie restriction (500 – 1,000 fewer calories than estimated as necessary for weight maintenance)
- Regular physical activity
- Frequent participant contact

Participants in this type of program have demonstrated an average weight reduction of 5 – 7% of body weight and successful long-term maintenance of their weight loss. Unfortunately, delivering this type of program is challenging since it is labor and time intensive. Most third-party payers do not cover medical nutrition therapy visits adequately enough to achieve weight loss goals through this type of program.

Risks and Benefits of a Low-Carbohydrate Diet for Weight Loss
The recommended daily allowance for digestible carbohydrate is 130 grams/day. This is based on the estimated need for glucose as fuel for the brain and to meet the dietary needs for fiber, vitamins and minerals found in carbohydrate foods. People on diets too low in carbohydrate are missing important nutrients that come from a balanced diet.

Two studies showed that subjects on low-carbohydrate diets lost more weight at 6 months than those on low-fat diets. However, at 1 year, weight loss between the two groups was roughly the same, with both demonstrating modest weight loss at that point.

Other studies demonstrate that low-carbohydrate diets have a favorable effect on triglycerides and HDL-C and are associated with a greater decrease in A1C in subjects with type 2 diabetes. On the other hand, LDL-C was significantly higher in these subjects.

The American Diabetes Association (ADA) recognizes the conflicting findings of this research and states that more study is needed to determine the long-term safety and efficacy of low-carbohydrate diets in people with diabetes.

Nutritional Considerations during Pregnancy

Nutritional goals during pregnancy include achieving normoglycemia and preventing ketosis. Tight glycemic control during pregnancy reduces the risk for serious perinatal complications and improves maternal health-related quality of life.

Weight loss during pregnancy is generally not recommended. Hypocaloric diets in obese women with gestational diabetes (GDM) can result in ketosis. However, a carefully monitored, moderate reduction in calories to achieve glycemic control is sometimes appropriate.

The diet for gestational diabetes is carbohydrate-controlled while meeting the nutritional needs for maternal and fetal health. The diet is individualized based upon body weight, glucose levels, ketone levels and use of insulin. The daily carbohydrate allowance during pregnancy should be at least 175 grams distributed throughout the day in 3 small to moderate-sized meals and 2 – 4 snacks. Evening snacks are sometimes required to prevent ketosis overnight. If the patient uses insulin, carbohydrate intake must be consistent to avoid hypoglycemia.

Regular physical activity can help lower plasma glucose concentrations and prevent excessive weight gain during pregnancy.

Exercise

Benefits of Physical Activity
Exercise improves glycemic control and lowers risk for cardiovascular disease and mortality. It can also prevent or delay the onset of diabetes in people at high risk.
Specific benefits of exercise include:
- Decreases insulin resistance
- Lowers fasting and postprandial glucose concentrations
- Improves uptake of glucose by muscle tissue
- Increases fat metabolism
- Increases cardiac output
- Helps with weight loss and maintenance of weight loss*
- Reduces BMI
- Decreases blood pressure by about 5 – 10 mmHg
- Modestly increases HDL cholesterol
- Modestly decreases triglyceride level
- Helps alleviate stress, depression and anxiety

*Following weight loss, regular exercise has been shown to be the primary predictor of maintaining the loss."

Effect of Exercise on Insulin Sensitivity
During the post-exercise period, there is increased uptake of glucose by the muscles mediated by increased insulin sensitivity of the muscular receptors. While insulin secretion decreases during exercise, the increased insulin sensitivity more than compensates for this, resulting in a lowering of the blood glucose concentration. This often results in decreased need for medications by people with diabetes who exercise regularly.

The favorable effect of exercise on insulin sensitivity is additive when exercise is performed daily. Depending upon the duration and intensity of the activity, the insulin-sensitizing effect lasts for 24 –72 hours following an exercise session. Therefore, to optimize the benefits of exercise, it is recommended that no more than 2 days pass between sessions.

Both aerobic and resistance exercise affect insulin sensitivity to about the same degree. There is evidence that insulin sensitivity following resistance exercise may last somewhat longer.

Effect of Exercise on Weight Loss
Exercise has long been recognized as an integral part of successful weight loss programs. However, exercise alone, without modification of diet or behavior, tends to result in only modest weight loss of approximately 4 – 5 pounds on average. Higher volume exercise regimens, such as 1 hour daily of moderate intensity aerobic exercise, have the most beneficial effect on weight loss.

For people with diabetes, the health benefits of exercise are greatest with regard to improved glycemic control and cardiovascular health but less pronounced with regard to weight loss. The greatest effect of exercise on weight loss seems to be in maintaining the loss over time. It has been found that people who have been able to maintain larger loss of weight for a year or more typically engage in about 7 hours per week of moderate to vigorous exercise.

Aerobic Exercise in Type 2 Diabetes
Aerobic exercise has been shown to decrease A1C results in people with type 2 diabetes regardless of weight loss. Increased aerobic fitness is also associated with significantly lower rates of cardiovascular disease and mortality.

While the recommendation for an activity program should be individualized, a target of at least 150 minutes of moderate aerobic activity per week is advised for most people with diabetes. Those who are already active can gain further benefits by increasing the intensity of their exercise.

Alternatively, 90 minutes of vigorous aerobic exercise per week can meet the activity requirement for people with type 2 diabetes. The exercise should be distributed over 3 days per week and no more than 2 consecutive days should elapse between exercise sessions.

Greater reduction in cardiovascular risk can be attained by performing at least 4 hours of moderate to vigorous aerobic and/or resistance exercise per week. Larger amounts of such exercise are also associated with maintenance of weight loss over the long-term.

Resistance Training in Type 2 Diabetes
Resistance training is a recommended part of the fitness program for people with type 2 diabetes. This type of exercise increases insulin sensitivity to the same degree as aerobic activity. It is especially beneficial to older adults, who are at risk for decline in muscle mass. Studies show that a resistance training regimen can lower A1C values in people with type 2 diabetes.

There is insufficient evidence to conclude that resistance exercise increases the risk for stroke, myocardial ischemia or retinal hemorrhage in people with type 2 diabetes. The American Diabetes Association (ADA) has concluded that high-intensity resistance training is safe for these individuals, even those with cardiovascular risk factors.

ADA recommendations call for resistance exercise 3 times per week in people with type 2 diabetes, who have no contraindications to such exercise. The exercises should target all major muscle groups and progress to 3 sets of 8 – 10 repetitions. The amount of weight used should be that which cannot be lifted more than 8 – 10 times.

Evaluation Prior to Exercise Program

It is generally safe to recommend a physical activity program of brisk walking to most people with type 2 diabetes without having them undergo cardiac stress testing. Those with predisposing risks such as severe neuropathy, either autonomic or peripheral, and preproliferative or proliferative retinopathy require more thorough evaluation.

For patients who plan to start an exercise program more vigorous than brisk walking, an assessment of cardiovascular risk factors is advised. The recommendation about when to perform exercise stress testing is controversial. American Diabetes Association (ADA) guidelines suggest that the clinical judgment of the healthcare provider should guide the decision about whether to perform cardiac stress testing. Examples of patients appropriate for the test include:

- Previously sedentary individuals with moderate to high risk for cardiovascular disease
- Those with concurrent autonomic neuropathy, peripheral vascular disease or microvascular disease
- Those with type 2 diabetes for longer than 10 years
- Those with type 1 diabetes for longer than 15 years if age 35 years or older

Exercise Precautions Type 1 Diabetes with Hyperglycemia

Hyperglycemia and ketosis can worsen if a person with type 1 diabetes initiates exercise while blood glucose is greater than 250 mg/dl and ketones are present. These clients should be advised to avoid exercise until blood glucose improves and ketones are absent.

If a client with type 1 diabetes has blood glucose of 250 – 300 mg/dl following overconsumption of carbohydrate and ketones are negative, exercise is probably safe. The absence of ketones signals that the person is not insulin-deficient at that time and the risk for ketosis is small.

If a client with type 1 diabetes has blood glucose greater than 300 mg/dl, it is prudent to delay exercise even in the absence of ketones.

Sometimes a person with type 1 diabetes experiences an acute rise in blood glucose following intense exercise, such as engaging in competitive sports. In this case, additional insulin should not be administered because its action will coincide with the increased insulin sensitivity that follows exercise.

Exercise Precautions for Type 2 Diabetes with Hyperglycemia

While people with type 1 diabetes are usually advised to delay exercise when hyperglycemia and ketones are present, this is usually not necessary for people with type 2 diabetes because they do not have a risk for severe insulin deficiency.

If a person with type 2 diabetes has a blood glucose level greater than 300 mg/dl, it is not necessary to advise them to abstain from exercise at that time, especially if they are in a postprandial state. As long as the person is not severely insulin deficient, increasing physical activity is likely to decrease blood glucose levels. If ketones are negative, insulin deficiency is not present.

The client should be advised to remain well-hydrated during exercise, especially when blood glucose is high. If ketones are present in the hyperglycemic client with type 2 diabetes, strenuous exercise should be avoided.

Exercise Program That Optimizes Fitness Level and Glycemic Response

At least 150 minutes of moderate to vigorous exercise per week is recommended. For optimal insulin sensitization, exercise should occur at least every other day on at least 3 nonconsecutive days.

For weight loss, more frequent exercise (e.g., 5 – 7 days per week) is needed.

For minimum health conditioning, 700 calories should be expended per week on exercise. Expending 2,000 calories per week yields maximum health and fitness benefits. There is little evidence to suggest that expending more than 2,000 calories per week on exercise substantially increases health and fitness benefits.

Intensity of exercise should be 50 – 85% of maximal age-adjusted heart rate. A target heart rate in that range is selected based upon the results of exercise stress testing or the individual's fitness level, age, duration of diabetes and presence of complications and comorbidities. In the absence of stress testing, maximal age-adjusted heart rate can be estimated by subtracting the client's age from 220.

Modifications to Exercise Program for Clients with Microvascular Complications

Proliferative or severe nonproliferative retinopathy – Clients should be instructed to avoid vigorous aerobic or resistance exercises to prevent vitreous hemorrhage and retinal detachment.

Peripheral neuropathy – Clients who have lost protective sensation in the lower extremities should be advised to avoid exercises that increase the risk for skin breakdown, joint injury and Charcot fracture. At the very least, protective and well-fitting shoes and socks should be worn at all times. In cases of severe loss of protective sensation, non-weight-bearing activities such as cycling or swimming are recommended.

Autonomic neuropathy – This poses risk for decreased cardiac response to exercise, postural hypotension, silent angina and impaired thirst sensation. These clients should undergo thorough cardiac evaluation before being recommended an exercise program.

Microalbuminuria – Exercise can increase urinary protein excretion but studies have not confirmed that exercise accelerates decline in kidney function. Therefore, the presence of microalbuminuria should not limit exercise. However, the cardiovascular status of microalbuminuric individuals should be considered since microalbuminuria and nephropathy are associated with increased cardiovascular risk.

Appropriate Exercise Program for Peripheral Vascular Disease

Intermittent claudication is PVD-related ischemic pain resulting from an inadequate oxygen supply to the muscles of the lower extremities. The pain is exacerbated by walking and alleviated by rest. Although it causes discomfort, a walking program is usually recommended to increase collateral circulation and improve condition. However, when the person has pain at rest or during the night, the degree of PVD is severe and a walking program is contraindicated.

The walking program is usually developed to provide intervals of activity and rest. The client is instructed to walk at a low intensity and to continue walking through low to moderate pain. Distraction techniques such as listening to music or talking to a partner can help. The client should rest when pain begins to elevate from moderate to intense.

Benefits from the interval exercise program are optimized when the client participates every day and engages in weight-bearing exercise.

Prevent Exercise-Induced Hypoglycemia

For individuals taking insulin or insulin secretagogues, blood glucose should be monitored before exercise and additional carbohydrate consumed if results are less than 100 mg/dl. Risk for hypoglycemia is especially high when injected insulin is at its peak action or exercise is prolonged.

For those not treated with insulin or secretagogues, exercise-induced hypoglycemia is rare. Updated American Diabetes Association (ADA) guidelines indicate that supplemental carbohydrate is not needed prior to exercise, even if blood glucose is less than 100 mg/dl when:
- Treating diabetes by lifestyle modification alone
- Using metformin, alpha-glucosidase inhibitors or thiazolidinediones without insulin or secretagogues

The risk of exercise-induced hypoglycemia associated with the amylin analog pramlintide or the incretin mimetic exenatide has not been studied. The ADA suggests that neither drug has high potential for causing exercise-induced hypoglycemia when used alone or in combination with metformin or a thiazolidinedione. If these medications are taken with insulin or a secretagogue, supplemental carbohydrate would be needed prior to exercise when blood glucose is below 100 mg/dl.

Post-Exercise, Late-Onset Hypoglycemia and Preventive Measures

Post-exercise, late-onset hypoglycemia (PEL) is exercise-induced low blood glucose that occurs 4 or more hours after exercise. It happens most commonly to people having type 1 diabetes, but anyone using insulin or insulin secretagogues is at risk. The risk is increased after exercising at moderate to intense levels for more than 30 minutes.

Physiologically, PEL is the result of exercise-related increases in glucose utilization and insulin sensitivity and the replenishment of glycogen stores post-exercise.

Clients who use insulin or insulin secretagogues should be educated about the risk for PEL and be instructed to watch for signs of impending hypoglycemia beyond the immediate post-exercise period. Adjustments to insulin can be made to avoid having peak action occur during the post-exercise period. Another option to prevent PEL is to have the client increase carbohydrate consumption after exercise. Clients at risk for PEL should not exercise prior to bedtime to prevent nocturnal hypoglycemia.

Insulin Injection Technique Affects

Insulin Absorption during Exercise

It is important to ensure that insulin is injected into the subcutaneous fat layer and to avoid intramuscular injection. Muscle contractions can hasten the absorption of insulin into the circulation and injecting into muscle increases the risk for exercise-induced hypoglycemia.

In the past, it was recommended to avoid injecting insulin into the part of the body involved in exercise. For example, injecting into the arm would have been recommended if the person was planning to jog or walk.

More recent research has indicated that this practice does not decrease the risk for exercise-induced hypoglycemia in the person taking insulin injections. Exercise increases insulin absorption no matter the site of injection, so exercise always increases the risk for hypoglycemia in these clients. To avoid hypoglycemia, they should decrease or adjust the insulin dose so that peak action does not coincide with the planned exercise period.

Carbohydrate Replacement during Exercise
If the person does not use insulin or an insulin secretagogue, carbohydrate replacement during exercise is usually not required since the risk for hypoglycemia is low.

For those using insulin, the best strategy is to reduce the dose or make adjustments so that peak insulin action does not coincide with exercise. When exercise occurs during the postprandial period, 1 –3 hours after a meal, carbohydrate supplementation may not be needed.

Carbohydrate supplementation may be needed to prevent hypoglycemia when exercise is unplanned or insulin adjustments are not possible. Blood glucose monitoring before, during and after exercise helps determine the individual's glycemic response to exercise and the need for supplementation.

For moderate exercise of 30 –60 minutes duration, 15 extra grams of carbohydrate is often appropriate.

For high-intensity exercise or exercise lasting for more than an hour, 30 –50 grams of additional carbohydrate may be needed for each hour of activity.

Oral Medications for Type 2 Diabetes

While the American Diabetes Association (ADA) recommends starting with metformin at the onset of type 2 diabetes, individual characteristics may alter the decision.

Liver and kidney function must be tested before starting any oral diabetes medication.

Metformin is not used when glomerular filtration rate (GFR) is less than 30 and/or serum creatinine is greater than 1.5 mg/dl in men or greater than 1.4 mg/dl in women.

When renal function is decreased, the risk for hypoglycemia is greater with the use of insulin secretagogues.

When the alanine aminotransferase (ALT) level is elevated above 2.5 times normal, the use of metformin and thiazolidinediones is contraindicated. Metformin is contraindicated in clients who drink alcohol excessively or engage in binge drinking. Thiazolidinediones are contraindicated in people with heart failure and severe cardiac disease. Metformin should be used with caution in these clients.

Glucose toxicity usually requires insulin prior to initiation of oral medications. Signs of glucose toxicity include prolonged hyperglycemia, A1C > 9% and possibly ketones.

Physiological Effects of Insulin

Insulin is a hormone secreted by the beta cells of the Islets of Langerhans in the pancreas.

Actions of insulin on body tissues include:
- Augments protein synthesis by promoting the entry of amino acids into the cells
- Promotes utilization of glucose for energy by stimulating its entry into the cells
- Enhances storage of unused glucose as glycogen in muscle and liver cells
- Enhances the storage of fat and prevents the use of fat breakdown for energy
- Impedes glycogenolysis, the making of glucose from glycogen stored in muscle and liver cells
- Impedes the formation of glucose from amino acids and other non-carbohydrate sources

Counter-regulatory hormones antagonize the hypoglycemic effects of insulin. They include glucagon, epinephrine, norepinephrine, growth hormone and cortisol.

Classifications of Insulin

Insulin type	Examples	Onset of action	Peak action	Duration of action	Teaching
Rapid-acting	Lispro Aspart	5 – 15 min	30 – 90 min	Less than 5 hours	Inject less than 15 minutes before eating. Injecting too early can cause profound hypoglycemia.
Short-acting	Regular Novolin R Humulin R	30 min	2 – 4 hours	5 – 8 hours	Like rapid-acting, is used as a bolus insulin to provide post-prandial glucose control.
Inter-mediate-acting	NPH Novolin N Humulin N	1 – 2 hours	4 – 10 hours	10 – 18 hours	Cloudy insulin; gently roll and rotate vial prior to filling syringe to resuspend particles.
Long-acting	Glargine Lantus Detemir Levemir	1 – 2 hours	None	Up to 24 hours	Do not mix in same syringe with other insulins.

Rapid-Acting Insulins

Rapid-acting insulins are given as bolus doses to provide post-meal blood glucose control. They include lispro and aspart insulin. They are usually used in place of Regular insulin and have shorter onset, peak and duration times.

Rapid-acting insulin begins to work in 5 – 15 minutes after injection. Clients should be cautioned to avoid injecting this type of insulin too early since profound hypoglycemia can result, especially with lispro. However, when compared with Regular insulin, both lispro and aspart have a lower overall risk for hypoglycemia.

Peak action for rapid-acting insulin is 1 – 2 hours. Duration is usually less than 5 hours. The injection of aspart insulin into the abdominal subcutaneous tissue has been shown to shorten the duration of its action time.

The rapid-acting insulins are suitable for multiple daily injections and for use with the insulin pump.

Long-Acting Insulins

Long-acting insulins include glargine and detemir. They are options for basal insulin therapy and should provide about 50% of the daily insulin requirement continuously over 24 hours. Long-acting insulin is often used in combination with bolus insulin or oral agents that provide postprandial blood glucose control.

Long-acting insulin can be given once or twice daily. When administered once daily, the dose is usually given at bedtime. It should always be given at the same time each day.

Long-acting insulins have a "peakless" action and therefore pose a lower risk for hypoglycemia than insulins with shorter action times. The risks for nocturnal hypoglycemia and weight gain are lower in people with type 2 diabetes who use long-acting insulin as compared to those who use NPH.

Patients using long-acting insulin should be instructed that the insulin is not to be mixed in the same syringe with other types of insulin.

Starting Dose for Insulin Therapy

Type 1 diabetes
Daily insulin requirements are usually between 0.5 – 1.0 units per kilogram of body weight. Requirements can be much higher during periods of illness or metabolic instability. During the "honeymoon phase," when some endogenous insulin is still being produced, injected daily insulin requirements are usually 0.2 – 0.6 units/kg of body weight.

Type 2 diabetes
There is more variability in the starting does of insulin for people with type 2 diabetes. The decision is based upon body weight, degree of insulin deficiency, suspected insulin resistance, glycemic goals and concurrent use of oral antidiabetic agents. Oral medications are often continued while insulin is added to the regimen.

For a single daily injection of basal insulin, 10 – 20 units per day is a common starting dose. Because of insulin resistance, initial starting dose relative to body weight is usually higher for type 2 diabetes, often 0.7 – 2.5 units/kg body weight daily.

Injection Regimen

Single and 2-dose daily insulin regimens can be utilized as monotherapy or in combination with oral antidiabetic agents in type 2 diabetes.

<u>Single daily injection</u>
- Contraindicated for type 1 diabetes
- Used when dose requirement is less than 30 units/day
- Administered in the morning or at bedtime using intermediate or long-acting insulin
- Intermediate-acting insulin could be mixed with rapid or short-acting insulin.
- Often administered at bedtime to improve fasting blood glucose or to suppress nocturnal glucose production by the liver

<u>Two-injection regimen</u>
- Administered before breakfast and in the evening, either before dinner or at bedtime
- May include 2 doses of intermediate or long-acting insulin only, or mixed intermediate and rapid or short-acting insulin at either or both injection times
- Typically, two-thirds of the total daily dose is given at the morning injection and one-third in the evening.

Intensive Insulin Therapy

Intensive insulin therapy includes 3 or more injections per day. Glycemic control is optimized when a basal bolus regimen mimics the physiologic profile of insulin secretion as closely as possible.

Basal insulin is intermediate or long-acting insulin which provides an ongoing low level of insulin to provide for basic metabolic needs. Bolus insulin is rapid or fast-acting insulin that is given to control post-meal blood glucose.

Examples of 3 and 4 daily-injection regimens include:
- Bolus insulin given before each meal
- Bolus insulin before each meal and basal insulin at bedtime
- Bolus insulin given before breakfast and lunch and basal insulin given at bedtime
- Bolus regimen with intermediate-acting insulin before breakfast + bolus insulin before the evening meal + intermediate-acting insulin at bedtime

When intermediate-acting insulin is given in the morning, bolus insulin should NOT be given at lunchtime, as the peak times for both insulins would coincide and could cause profound hypoglycemia.

Storage and Preparation of Insulin

Insulin vials that are currently in use can be stored at room temperature for the number of days that the manufacturer specifies, as long as room temperature remains between 36° and 86° F. Vials of insulin not in current use should be stored in a refrigerator and used by the printed expiration date. The client should always have a spare bottle of each type of insulin that he or she is using.

Care should be taken to avoid vigorous agitation of the insulin vial, as this can cause loss of potency.

Prior to drawing an injection, the client should inspect the insulin for signs of degradation such as clumping, frosting, precipitation or change in clarity or color. Rapid and fast-acting insulins, as well as glargine, should remain clear. Intermediate-acting insulin should remain uniformly cloudy without clumping.

In situations where a client has otherwise unexplained loss of glycemic control, reduction in insulin potency should be considered.

Mixing Two Types of Insulin in Same Syringe

Rapid-acting and regular insulin are drawn into the syringe before intermediate-acting insulin to avoid protamine contamination of the clear insulin. Glargine should never be mixed with another type of insulin.

Some mixtures come premixed by the manufacturer in predetermined ratios. An example is Humulin 70/30 which includes 70% NPH plus 30% regular insulin. While convenient, these mixtures have the disadvantage of decreasing the flexibility and fine-tuning of the regimen. They are most appropriately used with clients who need a simple regimen or who have cognitive or functional issues that impair their ability to mix insulin.

Prefilling syringes is acceptable if guidelines to protect the potency of the insulin are followed. Regular and NPH insulins can be mixed and stored in the refrigerator for 1 month. The syringes should be stored vertically with the needle pointing up to prevent the suspended insulin particles from clogging the needle.

Safety Precautions with Insulin Syringes

Clients using insulin should be carefully instructed that insulin syringes are manufactured in different sizes, according to the capacity of insulin they can hold. This can affect the value of the markings on the syringe used for measuring the insulin. For example, a 0.3 cc (30 unit) or 0.5 cc (50 unit) syringe has measurement marks in 1-unit increments, whereas a 1.0 cc (100 unit) syringe has measurement markings in 2-unit increments. When a client switches from one type of syringe to another, there is the risk that he or she will assume the measurement marks are the same for both syringes; this could lead to potentially dangerous dosing errors.

Insulin syringes should never be shared with another person.

Because bending or breaking needles increases the risk for needle-stick injury, these practices should be discouraged.

Educators should instruct clients on the appropriate disposal of medical sharps waste in compliance with their local ordinances.

Reuse of Insulin Syringes and Needles

Manufacturers of disposable needles and syringes recommend single use only. The American Diabetes Association (ADA) neither encourages nor prohibits needle and syringe reuse but provides guidelines for those who choose to reuse for convenience or economic reasons.

Personal hygiene will help reduce risk for infection related to using unsterile needles. Insulin is manufactured with bacteriostatic additives that are active against common skin contaminants, but the used needle may carry bacteria. Those who are immunocompromised should not reuse needles.

Guidelines for needle reuse include:
- Discard needle when it is visibly dull or damaged.
- Discard needle if it comes into contact with any environmental surface.
- Cap the needle to be reused after each use.
- Store the syringe at room temperature.
- Do not clean the needle with alcohol or any other disinfectant. This will remove the silicone coating that makes the injection more comfortable.
- Inspect injection sites for signs of infection or lipodystrophy.

Administering an Insulin Injection

Routine insulin injections should be made into subcutaneous tissue. Most people can accomplish this by grasping a fold of skin and injecting at a 90-degree angle. If a person is very thin, injecting at a 45-degree angle is advised. Shorter needles are also available.

Aspiration of the needle to check for blood is no longer considered necessary.

When using an insulin pen, the needle should remain embedded within the tissue and the plunger depressed for at least 5 seconds to ensure complete delivery of insulin from the device.

Air bubbles should be removed from the filled syringe to ensure proper insulin dose.

When clear fluid escapes the puncture site, pressure should be applied for 5 – 8 seconds. Rubbing the site is not advised. If it is suspected that a significant portion of the insulin has been lost due to leakage, blood glucose should be monitored within a few hours.

Injecting insulin at room temperature decreases the risk for a painful injection.

Metformin

Metformin prevents high blood glucose primarily by decreasing glucose dumping from the liver. A secondary effect is that it decreases insulin resistance.

The dosage range is 500 – 2,550 mg/day.

The most common side effects are gastrointestinal. These include nausea, bloating, gas, diarrhea and metallic taste in the mouth. They are more common with higher doses and in the first 2 weeks of therapy.

Metformin is contraindicated in patients with decreased renal function. Metformin should not be prescribed in those with a glomerular filtration rate less than 30, in men with serum creatinine greater than 1.5 mg/dl or women with serum creatinine greater than 1.4 mg/dl.

Metformin should not be used in people who drink more than 2 alcoholic beverages a day or engage in binge drinking.

Caution is advised when there is concurrent heart failure, dehydration, acidosis, NPO status or pending iodine radio contrast studies.

Patient Education for Metformin

- Take the medication with food to reduce risk for gastrointestinal side effects.
- If gastrointestinal side effects are severe, call your healthcare provider.
- The medication takes up to 1 month to reach maximum effectiveness.
- Use caution when drinking alcohol. Drinking in excess can cause a serious and life-threatening condition called lactic acidosis. Consult with your healthcare provider to ascertain if moderate alcohol consumption (less than 2 drinks per day) is safe for you.
- Stop taking metformin if you are not eating and drinking or become dehydrated.
- Stop taking metformin on the day of surgery or when having studies using radio contrast dye.
- This medication increases chances for becoming pregnant when it is prescribed to treat polycystic ovary syndrome. Discuss birth control options with your healthcare provider.
- Always carry medical identification stating that you have diabetes.

Sulfonylurea Medications

Sulfonylureas include glipizide, glyburide and tolazamide. They work by stimulating the pancreas to produce more insulin. They are only effective in people who maintain some beta cell function.

The most common side effect is hypoglycemia. The risk for this is greatest in the first few months of starting the medication. To prevent hypoglycemia, the patient should check blood glucose regularly, avoid delaying or missing meals and avoid drinking alcohol.

Other side effects include weight gain, sun sensitivity, headache and nausea.

Liver and kidney function should be tested prior to starting the sulfonylureas. If either function is low, the risk for hypoglycemia is increased. Exercise caution when prescribing to the elderly, who often have decreased liver and kidney function as well as a higher risk for hypoglycemic unawareness. Those with adrenal or pituitary insufficiency are also at higher risk for hypoglycemia when taking sulfonylureas.

People with severe sulfa allergies may not be able to take sulfonylurea medications.

Thiazolidinedione Medications

TZDs include pioglitazone and rosiglitazone. They work by increasing the insulin sensitivity of liver and skeletal tissues and by suppressing glucose production by the liver.

Side effects include weight gain, mild to moderate edema, bone fractures in women and upper respiratory symptoms.

When used alone, these agents do not cause hypoglycemia. However, when used with a sulfonylurea or insulin, risk may be increased.

TZDs have a black box warning that they may cause or exacerbate congestive heart failure (CHF) in some patients and are contraindicated in people with class III and IV heart failure. The manufacturer of rosiglitazone advises against prescribing this medication for any patient who uses nitrates or insulin, as these drug combinations have been associated with increased risk for cardiac problems.

TZDs are associated with rare cases of idiosyncratic hepatocellular damage. TZDs are used with caution in people with hepatic dysfunction. Serum transaminase should be checked every 2 months during first year of therapy and periodically thereafter.

Patient Education for Thiazolidinediones
Notify a healthcare provider immediately if edema, sudden weight gain, shortness of breath or other signs of fluid retention develop.

TZDs may induce ovulation in premenopausal women with insulin resistance. If applicable, discuss family planning and birth control with a healthcare provider.

It may take several weeks of therapy to realize optimal effect.

Drug effectiveness and risk for side effects are not altered by food. Take with or without food.

If using with insulin or a sulfonylurea, there is an increased risk for hypoglycemia. Monitor blood glucose regularly and be prepared to treat hypoglycemia with a fast-acting carbohydrate.

Do not take TZDs if you are pregnant or breastfeeding.

Always carry medical identification stating that you have diabetes.

Dipeptidyl Peptidase-4 Inhibitor Medications

DPP-4 inhibitors include sitagliptin and saxagliptin.

DPP-4 is an enzyme that rapidly inactivates the incretin hormones. Incretins are digestive hormones that are released from the small intestine after eating in response to the post-meal rise in blood glucose. They lower blood sugar by stimulating insulin release and by decreasing glucagon production in the pancreas. The DPP-4 inhibitors prolong active incretin levels, allowing for increased insulin action following the post-meal rise in blood glucose.

The most common side effects of DPP-4 inhibitors are upper respiratory infection, urinary tract infection and headache. They are unlikely to cause hypoglycemia because they do not work well when blood glucose is low.

These medications may be used in patients with renal issues when guidelines for dosage adjustments are followed.

Alpha-Glucosidase Inhibitor Medications

AGIs include acarbose and miglitol. They work by reducing the rate of starch digestion and slowing its absorption through the small intestine, thus lowering post-meal blood glucose levels.

The most common side effects of AGIs are abdominal pain, diarrhea and flatulence. Side effects can be minimized by starting with a low dose and titrating upward.

When used alone, AGIs do not cause hypoglycemia. However, patients also using insulin or a sulfonylurea remain at risk for hypoglycemia. When taking these medications concurrently, patients require special instructions for treating hypoglycemia since the AGIs block the absorption of complex sugars. Only glucose and lactose are effective in treating hypoglycemia in patients who take AGIs.

To be effective, AGIs must be taken with the first bite of the meal.

AGIs are contraindicated in inflammatory bowel disease, cirrhosis, malabsorption disorders, pregnancy and lactation. They are not recommended in patients with serum creatinine greater than 2.0 mg/dl or with creatinine clearance of less than 25 ml/min.

Patient Education for AGIs
To be effective, acarbose and miglitol must be taken with the first bite of food at the meal. Initially, the medication may be used only once a day to minimize gastrointestinal side effects. GI side effects should lessen over a few weeks. If the low initial dose is tolerated, it will be titrated upward until the desired therapeutic effect is reached. By that point, AGI therapy is usually being taken at all three meals each day.

Patients using an AGI concurrently with a sulfonylurea or insulin are at risk for hypoglycemia from the latter two medications. If hypoglycemia occurs while using an AGI, most standard treatments will not be effective since the medication blocks the absorption of complex sugars through the small intestine. The only types of carbohydrate that will be effective are lactose (milk) and glucose (usually tablets).

Carry medical identification that states you have diabetes.

Meglitinide Medications

Meglitinides include repaglinide and nateglinide. They work by stimulating the pancreas to promptly release insulin in a glucose-dependent fashion with a shorter duration of action than sulfonylureas.

Hypoglycemia is a potential side effect of meglitinides. However, the risk is significantly lower as compared to sulfonylureas. Other side effects are not common but may include gastrointestinal complaints, upper respiratory symptoms, back pain and arthralgia.

Meglitinides must be taken within 30 minutes of the meal (0 – 30 minutes). If a meal is skipped, the medication dose is to be withheld. For this reason, meglitinides may be a good choice for patients with erratic eating habits.

Meglitinides are normally started at a low dose and titrated upward until glycemic goals are met. These medications should be used cautiously in patients with impaired hepatic function. Cautious use is also recommended in any patient with increased risk for hypoglycemia, such as the elderly and those with impaired renal, adrenal or pituitary function.

Incretin Mimetic Medications

Incretin mimetics include exenatide and liraglutide. They mimic the action of the incretin hormones glucagon-like peptide-1 (GLP-1) and gastric inhibitory polypeptide (GIP), causing an increase in insulin secretion from the pancreas. They also delay gastric emptying, increasing satiety and promoting weight loss.

Incretin mimetics are distributed as prefilled pens to be given as a subcutaneous injection. Exenatide is given within 30 – 60 minutes prior to the morning and evening meals. Missed doses should not be administered after the meal. Exenatide is not labeled for use with insulin and is contraindicated in type 1 diabetes. Exenatide has been associated with pancreatitis and is contraindicated in patients with a history of this condition. The most common side effects are nausea, vomiting and diarrhea. Hypoglycemia can occur if exenatide is used in conjunction with a sulfonylurea.

Liraglutide carries a black box warning cautioning that thyroid tumors were observed in rodent tests of this medication. Liraglutide is not approved as a first-line medication. It is delivered as a once-daily subcutaneous injection.

Patient Education for Incretin Memetics
Exenatide and liraglutide are administered subcutaneously by injection into the abdomen, thigh or upper arm.

The injection should be given within 30 – 60 minutes of the meal, usually twice a day with exenatide and once a day with liraglutide. Do not administer after a meal. If a meal is missed, skip the dose.

Store the prefilled syringes in the refrigerator. Remove needle from pen after each use.

Gastrointestinal side effects are common. These can sometimes be alleviated by injecting the medication closer to the mealtime. Nausea frequently subsides with continued use.

The patient should report possible signs and symptoms of pancreatitis, such as persistent abdominal pain or vomiting.

Oral antibiotics and contraceptives should be taken 1 hour apart from incretin mimetics.

Always carry medical identification stating that you have diabetes.

Basal and Bolus Components of Insulin Pump

Although the pump is designed to provide both basal and bolus insulin, the only type of insulin used with the pump is rapid-acting, such as lispro or aspart.

The basal dose is programmed to deliver a constant supply of insulin at a low level. The basal dose can be set to vary for particular time periods throughout the day. For example, a patient having elevated early morning blood glucose may set the pump to deliver more insulin in the pre-waking and early morning hours. Basal rates are highly individualized and depend upon blood glucose patterns and usual activity level. Typically, 4 – 6 different basal rates are set for a 24-hour period.

Bolus rates are designed to correct for episodes of high blood glucose and to cover the anticipated carbohydrate load of a meal. The client pushes a button on the pump to deliver the bolus dose at the appropriate time.

Continuous Subcutaneous Insulin Infusion

Technical malfunction of the pump can cause interruptions in insulin delivery and may result in ketosis.

As with any insulin use, hypoglycemia is a risk. The risk for inflammation and infection at the catheter insertion site can be reduced by following good personal hygiene, careful hand washing and changing the site and tubing every 3 days. Changing the tubing at this interval also prevents clogging.

Tube and reservoir changes should be done early in the day to avoid undetected malfunction during sleep.

Consistently rotating insertion sites reduces the risk for lipodystrophy and maintains good absorption of the insulin.

The insulin pump should be removed when the client is undergoing X-rays, CT scans, MRIs or radiation therapy and the device should be kept out of these treatment areas.

Initial Dosing and Adjustment for Oral Medication

Sulfonylureas are initiated at the lowest dose and titrated upward until glycemic goals are attained or maximum dose is reached.

Meglitinide doses do not need titration. The initial and maintenance dose is normally 120 mg taken before each meal.

The biguanide dose usually starts at 500 mg per day for adults and 250 mg daily for children. Although normally subtherapeutic, the starting dose is low to minimize gastrointestinal side effects. Gradual increases are made about every 2 weeks.

Thiazolidinediones are typically started at a low dose and gradually titrated upward to achieve glycemic targets. Adjustments should be made every 8 – 12 weeks, as this much time is needed for the optimal benefit to be realized.

Alpha-glucosidase inhibitors are initiated at lower doses to minimize gastrointestinal effects. The initial dose is usually 25 mg with meals, starting with one meal per day, and increased to patient tolerance.

Dipeptidyl peptidase-4 (DPP-4) inhibitors have once-daily dosing that does not require titration. Dosage adjustments are made for patients with renal issues.

1700 Rule

The 1700 Rule assumes that only rapid-acting insulin is being used as a bolus to correct high blood glucose. If correcting with regular insulin, the 1500 Rule is used. There is no standard formula for safely correcting hyperglycemia with intermediate or long-acting insulin.

The 1700 Rule determines by approximately how many mg/dl the blood glucose will be lowered by 1 unit of insulin.

1. Add up total daily insulin dose. This includes rapid, short, intermediate and long-acting insulin.
Example: 10 units of aspart before each meal and 30 units of NPH at bedtime. Total daily dose = 60 units

2. Divide 1700 by the total daily dose.
Example: 1700 divided by 60 = 28

3. One unit of aspart will lower the blood glucose approximately 28 mg/dl.

4. If blood glucose is 210 mg/dl and the target is 100 mg/dl, the correction dose would be approximately 4 units of aspart.
Example: 210 – 100 = 110
110 divided by 28 = 3.93 (round to 4.0)

Medications That Interact with Diabetes Treatment

Medications that can raise blood glucose levels:
- Glucocorticoids, such as prednisone
- Thiazide diuretics, such as HCTZ
- Phenytoin
- Estrogen compounds
- Antipsychotics, such as clozapine, olanzapine and risperidone

Non-diabetes medications that can lower blood glucose:
- Some antibiotics, such as clarithromycin and levofloxacin
- Salicylates in large doses
- Ethanol (alcohol), especially if consumed without food

Medications that can raise blood pressure or interfere with effectiveness of blood pressure medications:
- Anti-inflammatory agents, such as ibuprofen
- Glucocorticoids
- Over-the-counter nasal decongestants and cold remedies
- Oral contraceptives
- Tricyclic antidepressants, such as nortriptyline

Medications that mask hypoglycemia
- Beta blockers, such as propranolol

Clients should be encouraged to keep an updated list of all their medications and to bring it to each appointment so that possible drug interactions can be detected.

Safety Issues Related to Herbs

An evaluation of the use of herbs should be included in the medication assessment. Although these are sold over-the-counter, there are potential safety issues with their use. These issues include:
- Gastrointestinal side effects such as diarrhea (dandelion), or fecal impaction (guar gum).
- Dosages are not well-established, increasing the risk for toxicity.
- Some have potential to raise blood glucose (ma huang, rosemary).
- Some have potential to lower blood glucose, thereby increasing risk for hypoglycemia in clients using insulin or secretagogues (fenugreek, ginseng, prickly pear/cactus).
- Some have the potential to raise blood pressure (ma huang, licorice).
- Some have potential for liver damage (chaparral, sassafras, comfrey).
- All have potential for interaction with other medications.
- Most herbs have not been adequately studied for safety and efficacy.
- They are not standardized for purity and strength.

Assessment of liver and kidney function is important for the client who uses herbs.

Many herbs are deemed unsafe for use during pregnancy.

Unproven Therapies

ADA criteria for deeming an alternative therapy to be safe and effective are that they must be approved by Food and Drug Administration (FDA) and be supported by at least 2 studies published in a scientific, peer-reviewed journal.

When clients are interested in using alternative therapies, the educator should help them evaluate the claims made by the product and identify the symptoms being targeted by the therapy. Clients should keep a journal of symptoms and their response following implementation of the therapy. Professional complementary care providers are available through the American Holistic Nurses Association and Healing Touch International.

Although not endorsed by the ADA, some alternative modalities that are potentially useful for diabetes are:
- Omega-3 and omega-6 fatty acids to improve lipid profile
- Alpha lipoic acid and capsaicin for symptoms of neuropathy
- Fenugreek seeds, chromium picolinate and psyllium to lower blood glucose

At one time, cinnamon was believed to lower blood glucose but several follow-up studies did not support this.

Severe Hypoglycemia

Severe hypoglycemia is defined as the level at which the patient requires the assistance of another person to treat the symptoms.

Risk factors for severe hypoglycemia include:
- Type 1 diabetes. About 2 – 4% of deaths in people with type 1 diabetes are due to hypoglycemia. In type 1 disease, the normal glucagon response to low blood glucose diminishes, leading to an increased risk for hypoglycemic unawareness.
- History of recurrent hypoglycemic episodes. The brain adapts to previous hypoglycemia by shifting the sympathetic nervous system response to a lower plasma glucose concentration. The result is an increased risk for severe hypoglycemia.
- Insulin excess. Inappropriate insulin dosing or increased insulin sensitivity can create insulin excess. People with type 2 diabetes using insulin may experience insulin excess if they also use insulin sensitizing medication at the wrong time or take the wrong dose.
- Alcohol consumption. Alcohol can inhibit gluconeogenesis and can lead to hypoglycemia, especially if the person is in a starved state.

Treatment of Severe Hypoglycemia

For people who are alert enough to follow instructions and can swallow, ingestion of 15 – 20 grams of oral carbohydrate is appropriate. This step can be repeated after 15 – 20 minutes if hypoglycemic symptoms persist or blood glucose remains below 70 mg/dl.

For people who are unconscious or cannot swallow, intravenous glucose or glucagon, delivered subcutaneously or intramuscularly, are the only treatment choices. No oral treatment should be administered to or placed buccally in people who are not alert enough to swallow.

Family members can be taught to administer glucagon to high-risk clients. It is most helpful with type 1 diabetes. Side effects, such as nausea, vomiting and headache, are common following glucagon injection.

Intravenous treatment for hypoglycemia is usually 10 – 25 grams of 50% dextrose administered over 1 – 3 minutes.

People treated with either glucagon or intravenous glucose should consume oral carbohydrate as soon as they are able to eat.

Treatment for Mild to Moderate Hypoglycemia

Hypoglycemia is usually defined as plasma glucose less than 70 mg/dl.

Clients should check blood glucose as soon as symptoms appear to verify hypoglycemia.

When testing for hypoglycemia, the blood sample should be taken from the fingertip. Blood samples from alternate sites, such as the forearm, are not appropriate for detecting hypoglycemia.

Treatment for hypoglycemia is 15 – 20 grams of oral carbohydrate for plasma glucose ranging from 51 – 70 mg/dl. For glucose of 50 mg/dl or less, 20 – 30 grams of oral carbohydrate should be initially consumed.

Blood glucose should be rechecked 15 minutes after taking the carbohydrate. The treatment is repeated if blood glucose remains below 70 mg/dl.

The treatment should be followed with a planned meal or with an additional snack if the meal is more than 1 hour away.

At Risk for Hypoglycemia

Clients using insulin and/or oral blood glucose lowering medications need to be aware of the peak action times for these medications. Other measures to prevent hypoglycemia include taking care to administer the proper dose of medication at the right time and to avoid delaying or missing meals.

Clients on insulin should have a glucagon kit available and have significant others who know where it is located and how to administer it.

Medical identification stating that the person has diabetes and is on insulin is critical, as this may prevent treatment delay in an emergency.

Clients should be instructed to initially treat symptoms of hypoglycemia with 15 – 20 grams of oral carbohydrate. Over-treatment with too much carbohydrate is to be avoided so that hyperglycemia does not occur later. If the initial treatment does not raise the blood glucose to more than 70 mg/dl after 15 minutes has passed, an additional 15 grams of carbohydrate should be consumed.

Carbohydrate, Protein and Fat Consumption in the Treatment of Hypoglycemia
The preferred treatment for hypoglycemia is prompt oral ingestion of 15 – 20 grams of glucose, which is available in tablet form and also found in carbohydrate foods. Examples of foods equal to 15 grams of carbohydrate appropriate for treatment of hypoglycemia include:
- 4 oz fruit juice
- 7 – 8 Life Savers
- 8 oz fat-free milk
- 1 Tbsp sugar, jelly or honey

Ten grams of oral glucose raises plasma glucose levels by about 40 mg/dl over 30 minutes, while 20 grams raises it approximately 60 mg/dl over 45 minutes.

Following oral glucose treatment, plasma glucose levels begin to fall after about 60 minutes. Therefore, blood glucose should be tested again at this point as additional treatment may be required.

Adding protein to the glucose treatment does not affect the acute glycemic response of the treatment, nor does it prevent later hypoglycemia.

Adding fat to the oral glucose treatment may slow and prolong the glycemic response.

Glycemic Goals for Hospitalized Patients

Research supports optimal glycemic control for hospitalized patients with diabetes, showing that this reduces morbidity, mortality, length of stay and hospital cost.

However, other recent studies indicate that tight glycemic control in critically ill patients can increase the risk for severe hypoglycemia and mortality.

The American Diabetes Association (ADA) provides the flowing guidelines for glycemic control in hospitalized patients:
- Critically ill patients. A plasma glucose range of 140 – 180 mg/dl is recommended for most critically ill patients. Insulin should be started at a threshold of no greater than 180 mg/dl.
- Non-critically ill patients. Pre-meal plasma glucose should be less than 140 mg/dl or less if this can be achieved safely. Random plasma glucose should remain at 180 mg/dl or less. For stable patients with previously tight glycemic control, lower targets may be established if deemed safe. Less strict goals may be appropriate for patients with severe comorbidities.

Diabetic Ketoacidosis

<u>Laboratory Values</u>
Laboratory values include:
- Elevated plasma glucose (often to greater than 300 mg/dl but lower values do not preclude diagnosis)
- Arterial pH less than 7.2
- Bicarbonate value less than 15 mEq/l
- Positive ketones

Infection precipitates about 40% of DKA cases. Another common cause is the omission of insulin on sick days. Many patients are unaware that they should continue taking insulin even if they are not eating due to illness.

Less common precipitating factors include myocardial infarction, trauma, stress and surgery. Certain medications, such as corticosteroids and thiazide diuretics, can precipitate DKA.

Use of the insulin pump can increase the risk for DKA. This is because the insulin pump infuses only rapid-acting insulin, which has a very short duration of action. In the event of pump malfunction, there is no longer-acting insulin on board, resulting in insulin deficiency.

<u>Pathophysiology of Diabetic Ketoacidosis</u>
Diabetic ketoacidosis (DKA) is a syndrome of hyperglycemia, ketosis, dehydration and electrolyte imbalance caused by insulin deficiency. It is most commonly associated with type 1 diabetes.

Many cases of DKA are precipitated by illness, infection or trauma. Omission of insulin doses is the second leading cause of DKA. Cardiovascular events, such as myocardial infarction, can also precipitate DKA.

Profound insulin deficiency results in:
- Decreased glucose uptake, leading to hyperglycemia
- Excessive protein degradation leading to increased hepatic glucose production, which in turn exacerbates hyperglycemia
- Increased action of counter-regulatory hormones, leading to:
  - Production of free fatty acids that change into ketone bodies, which precipitate acidosis when unbuffered.
  - Decrease in the effectiveness of insulin

Hyperglycemia leads to:
- Osmotic diuresis, causing fluid loss and electrolyte depletion
- Excretion of ketone bodies, leading to depletion of sodium, potassium, chloride and fluid

Symptoms of Hyperglycemia and Clinical Presentation of Diabetic Ketoacidosis
The classic symptoms of hyperglycemia are the "three polys" – polydipsia, polyuria and polyphagia. Polyphagia occurs after more prolonged periods of insulin deficiency, such as days to weeks.

Other symptoms of hyperglycemia are blurred vision, weakness, lethargy, headache, malaise and nausea.

The clinical presentation of DKA includes:
- Signs of dehydration. These signs may include orthostatic hypotension, which is a drop in systolic blood pressure of 20 mmHg after 1 minute of standing compared to a baseline measurement with the patient supine.
- Abdominal symptoms, such as vomiting or abdominal pain
- Hyperventilation manifested as deep, rapid Kussmaul respirations
- Acetone breath with a fruity odor
- Hypothermia, although patient may have a fever if illness precipitated DKA.
- Abdominal pain characterized by tenderness and guarding
- Depressed mental status, such as stupor and eventually coma in severe cases

DKA may progress slowly over days if caused by mild insulin insufficiency. It can progress rapidly in acute illness or from other causes of severe insulin deficiency.

Treatment and Management of DKA
In mild cases of DKA, assuming the patient is able to ingest fluids, oral rehydration on an outpatient basis may be appropriate. The patient should be able to ingest and retain 3 – 5 ounces of fluid per hour. Insulin supplementation is also required.

For moderate to severe DKA, immediate intravenous fluid replacement and correction of electrolyte imbalance is critical. Insulin replacement with fast or short-acting insulin is also required.

In the absence of cardiac or respiratory arrest, hypovolemia is the most critical concern. Fluid replacement not only corrects hypovolemia, but also decreases hyperglycemia. Hyperglycemia will persist as long as acidosis is present and if fluid replacement is inadequate.

Replacement of potassium is crucial due to the profound potassium depletion associated with DKA.

If infection is the precipitating cause of DKA, it must also be treated.

Patients with prior DKA require education on the causes and prevention, with emphasis on sick day management to prevent future episodes.

<u>Diabetic Ketoacidosis vs. Hyperosmolar Hyperglycemic State</u>
DKA and HHS are acute complications of hyperglycemia. Either can occur in patients with previously undiagnosed diabetes and evolve into a medical crisis. Illness and infections are precipitating factors for both conditions.

Both conditions involve insufficiency of available insulin coupled with a substantial increase in the counter-regulatory hormones. The fundamental differentiating factor is ketosis, which is absent in HHS.

The degree of hyperglycemia varies between the two conditions. DKA occurs at plasma glucose levels as low as 250 mg/dl, while the blood glucose is usually greater than 600 mg/dl in HHS.

Both can potentially produce life-threatening hypovolemia.

HHS occurs in type 2 diabetes, most commonly in the elderly. It has a slower onset and longer duration of symptoms. HHS causes a slow decline in mental status over days or weeks and has a higher mortality rate.

DKA occurs in younger patients with type 1 diabetes, with a more rapid onset. Symptoms are more acute and include Kussmaul respirations and severe abdominal pain.

Hyperosmolar Hyperglycemic State

HHS is an acute complication of hyperglycemia associated with type 2 diabetes. The syndrome includes:
- Profound dehydration
- Neurological manifestations
- The absence of ketosis

Characteristics of HHS include:
- It is most commonly seen in elderly people with type 2 diabetes. Living alone or in a situation of inadequate monitoring increases the risk. Decreased thirst sensation contributes to the risk.
- It has a slow, insidious onset, causing it to be overlooked in many cases.
- It can be confused with other conditions, such as stroke.
- The condition is often precipitated by illness.

Signs and symptoms include:
- Signs of dehydration, such as orthostatic hypotension and dry membranes
- Evidence of decreased mental function, such as lethargy and confusion
- Neurological signs that mimic cerebral vascular accident, such as hemiparesis and aphasia
- Hyperglycemia, usually with a blood glucose level greater than 600 mg/dl
- Abdominal pain that is mild and less marked than in diabetic ketoacidosis (DKA)
- No ketone bodies in blood or urine, except in small amounts in some cases

<u>Pathophysiology of the Hyperosmolar Hyperglycemic State</u>
HHS is a syndrome of severe hyperglycemia and profound dehydration that can occur in people with type 2 diabetes.

Ketosis is absent in HHS because there is usually enough insulin present to prevent the excessive fat metabolism that produces ketone bodies. In the absence of acidosis, the patient with developing HHS does not usually experience the acute abdominal symptoms found in diabetic ketoacidosis (DKA). Because the patient is less likely to seek medical attention, extremely high blood glucose levels can result.

As glucose builds in the blood, it produces a hyperosmolar state. This causes water to be pulled from body cells, including the brain cells, accounting for the appearance of neurological/cognitive signs and symptoms such as decreased mental status and seizures.

Because of the profound dehydration of HHS, rehydration is the first priority of emergency treatment, followed by the correction of electrolyte deficits.

<u>Treatment of the Hyperosmolar Hyperglycemic State</u>
Emergency treatment and inpatient admission are required to treat HHS.

Fluid replacement is the first priority. Initially, 0.9% normal saline is usually administered as rapidly as possible over the first hour followed by a less concentrated saline solution at slower rates over the ensuing hours. As blood glucose declines, 5% dextrose may be used. Fluid replacement is individualized based upon the patient's hydration and cardiovascular status. Care is taken to avoid fluid overload.

Insulin therapy is required, although correction of dehydration alone improves glucose levels. Insulin dosing is conservative since rapid reduction of blood glucose can cause cerebral edema.

Monitoring and correcting potassium is crucial due to profound potassium depletion that results from treating a hyperglycemic emergency.

If infection is the precipitating cause of HHS, it must be treated.

Patients with prior HHS require education on the causes and prevention, with emphasis on sick day management to prevent future episodes. The importance of maintaining adequate hydration should also be emphasized.

Chronic Complications of Diabetes

A1C – Check at least twice a year in clients with stable glycemic control. Perform the test quarterly if not meeting glycemic goals or if changing therapy.

Hypertension – Blood pressure should be measured at each routine medical visit. If blood pressure is greater than 130/80 mmHg, measure again on another day.

Dyslipidemia – Fasting lipid profile should be measured at least annually.

Smoking – Ask clients at each routine visit if they smoke and advise quitting if necessary.

Nephropathy – Test for microalbuminuria annually. Perform serum creatinine measurement at least once a year.

Retinopathy –Dilated eye exam is recommended for all people with diabetes annually but it can be less frequent if client has had one or more normal exams. All screening exams for retinopathy should be performed by an ophthalmologist or optometrist.

Foot – Perform comprehensive foot exam annually, including testing for loss of protective sensation.

Diabetic Retinopathy

Diabetic retinopathy can often be detected within 5 years of diagnosis of either type 1 or type 2 diabetes. Since type 2 diabetes can be present or undetected for years prior to diagnosis, a significant number of patients already have retinopathy at the time of diagnosis.

The development and progression of retinopathy is highly correlated with the duration of diabetes and the degree of glycemic control. Optimization of glucose control is imperative for lowering risk. Blood pressure control can significantly contribute to the prevention of retinopathy and in slowing its progression.

Other risk factors for retinopathy include:
- Hypertension
- Pregnancy*
- Smoking
- Genetic predisposition
- Hyperlipidemia
- Puberty
- Renal failure

*Women with diabetes who plan to become pregnant should be counseled on the increased risk for the development or progression of retinopathy related to pregnancy. Comprehensive eye exam by an optometrist or ophthalmologist should take place in the first trimester with close follow-up throughout pregnancy and postpartum.

Pathophysiology of Diabetes Retinopathy
Retinopathy results from damage to the microvasculature supplying the part of the eye responsible for focusing images and light.

Hyperglycemic damage causes small hemorrhages and blood leakage through the vessel walls. To compensate for the loss of normal blood flow from damaged vessels, new blood vessels develop (neovascularization). These new vessels are so fragile that they leak and bleed easily, causing adhesions between the retina and the vitreous. This leads to retinal traction and detachment followed by vitreous bleeding that causes blindness. Macular edema is an additional serious consequence of retinal vessel leakage.

In nonproliferative retinopathy, microaneurysms and other evidence of vessel leakage are seen on fundus exam. The client does not experience any changes in vision at this time. Nonproliferative retinopathy is staged from mild to very severe.

Proliferative retinopathy indicates that neovascularization has started and there is resulting impairment in vision. This can range to mild blurring to large blind spots in the fields of vision.

Treatment of Diabetic Retinopathy

Glycemic control is paramount in preventing retinopathy and for minimizing its progression. Smoking cessation and managing hypertension and dyslipidemia are also fundamental treatment measures.

Patients with any evidence of retinopathy should be promptly referred to an ophthalmologist.

Mild to moderate nonproliferative retinopathy requires only observation and optimization of glycemic, blood pressure and lipid control.

For proliferative retinopathy, laser photocoagulation therapy is indicated. This may also be indicated for some cases of severe to very severe nonproliferative retinopathy. Multiple outpatient treatment sessions are usually necessary. Most patients require anesthetic eye drops, although a local anesthetic injection may be available if needed.

Studies show that laser photocoagulation surgery is effective in preventing further vision loss, but not in restoring acuity that has already been lost. Some patients experience a small decline in acuity and peripheral vision following photocoagulation therapy, but this is generally offset by the preservation of central vision.

Surgical vitrectomy may be required in cases of retinal detachment or when hemorrhages do not resolve after laser surgery.

Other Ocular Complications

Blurred vision is a common symptom of hyperglycemia and is also common during periods of fluctuating glycemic control. It is a transient condition caused by osmotic changes in the eyeball. When this condition occurs, clients should postpone changes in eyeglass prescriptions until blood glucose has stabilized for 6 – 8 weeks.

Cataracts are more common in people with diabetes. They occur at a younger age and progress more aggressively than in people who do not have diabetes. They are easily detected on eye exam. They can be corrected with a minor outpatient surgery that replaces the clouded lens with an artificial one.

Open-angled glaucoma may not occur more frequently in diabetes. However, the risk for vision loss is greater when blood glucose control is suboptimal due to compromised circulation.

Ischemic optic neuropathy is optic nerve damage caused by microvascular impairment. It can cause irreversible loss of vision.

Sexual Dysfunction

Sexual dysfunction in diabetes is related to autonomic neuropathy. Up to 75% of men and 35% of women with diabetes experience difficulty with sexual functioning.

Erectile dysfunction is a common problem in men with diabetes. This is usually accompanied by loss of testicular pain sensation with pressure and loss of perineal sensation. Assessment includes ruling out other causes such as antihypertensive medications or psychological reasons. The patient and partner can be referred to a urologist or an impotence clinic. Treatments include surgical penile implants, suction devices that produce erection, prostaglandin injections and oral medications, such as sildenafil.

Manifestations of female sexual dysfunction in diabetes include decreased lubrication, delayed, blunted or absent arousal and absent orgasmic response. Referral to a gynecologist may be appropriate. Treatment includes application of vaginal lubricant and use of estrogen. Causes of female sexual dysfunction other than autonomic neuropathy could be depression or vaginal infection.

Sensory Neuropathy

Sensory neuropathy causes sensory deficits that usually begin in the distal portion of the lower extremities. The deficits sometimes progress to the distal upper extremities, in what is known as a "stocking-glove" distribution.

Identifying sensory neuropathy is a diagnosis of exclusion, although extensive testing to rule out other causes is not often necessary.

Assessment includes:
- Monofilament testing for loss of tactile sensation
- Testing for loss of vibratory sensation by applying a tuning fork at the distal first metatarsal head
- Checking temperature sensation by using the cool metal part of a reflex hammer or tuning fork on the skin and asking the patient to describe the temperature
- Testing position sensation by flexing and extending the big toes and asking the patient to describe the position

There are no treatments to reverse neuronal loss. Improved glycemic control and smoking cessation can slow or halt further progression of nerve damage. Palliative treatments for pain include medications such as tricyclic antidepressants, anticonvulsants and capsaicin cream.

Autonomic Neuropathies

Autonomic neuropathy has the potential to affect every system in the body. About 50% of people with diabetic peripheral neuropathy also have autonomic neuropathy.

The autonomic neuropathies and manifestations of each include:
- Neurogenic bladder – difficulty emptying bladder, dribbling, frequent bladder infections
- Sexual dysfunction – erectile dysfunction, decreased vaginal lubrication, absent orgasmic response

- Gastroparesis – early satiety, heartburn, anorexia, postprandial hypoglycemia
- Intestinal impairment – fecal incontinence, nocturnal diarrhea, constipation
- Orthostatic hypotension – drop in blood pressure from sitting position to standing; dizziness, lightheadedness, syncope
- Cardiac denervation* – fixed heart rate, silent myocardial infarction, abnormal cardiovascular response to exercise
- Hypoglycemic unawareness – lack of normal symptoms with low blood glucose
- Impaired insulin counter-regulation – "brittle diabetes" in type 1 diabetes
- Anhidrosis – failure to sweat; cracked, fissured heels
- Abnormal pupillary response to light – slow dilation of pupils

*Cardiovascular autonomic neuropathy is associated with significant morbidity and mortality.

Autonomic Neuropathy Affects on Gastrointestinal Tract
Because the entire gastrointestinal (GI) system has autonomic innervation, neuropathy may affect any part of it from the esophagus to the rectum.

Gastroparesis results in delayed emptying of stomach contents. It can interfere with the absorption of glucose and oral medications, leading to suboptimal glycemic control and unpredictable postprandial glycemic response.

Symptoms of gastroparesis include reflux, heartburn, anorexia, early satiety, nausea, vomiting and erratic blood glucose levels.

Referral to a gastroenterologist and dietitian are indicated for gastroparesis. Dietary measures include low-fat/low-fiber diet with multiple small meals. Medications that increase stomach motility, such as metoclopramide, are useful.

The most common lower-intestinal autonomic disorder is constipation. Adequate fiber in the diet along with good hydration and regular physical activity are recommended to treat and prevent constipation. Stool softeners, bulk laxatives (e.g., psyllium) and medications to increase intestinal motility are also used.

As with all complications of diabetes, optimal glucose control and smoking cessation are indicated for autonomic neuropathies affecting the GI system.

Autonomic Neuropathies That Affect Cardiovascular Function
Both sympathetic and parasympathetic nerves innervate the cardiovascular system and can be affected by neuropathy. This can affect heart rate, heart rhythm and blood pressure maintenance.

Mortality associated with cardiovascular autonomic neuropathy is estimated to be as high as 56% within 5 – 10 years of onset. Sudden death is associated with silent ischemia and cardiac arrhythmias.

Manifestations of autonomic neuropathy affecting the cardiovascular system include:
- Fixed heart rate
- Orthostatic hypotension
- Decreased cardiac response to exercise
- Absence or altered perception of cardiac ischemia

- Insufficient hemodynamic response to cardiovascular stressors such as surgery and infection
- Predisposition to cardiac arrhythmias

Interventions for orthostatic hypotension include:
- Prevention of falls
- Making position changes slowly
- Use of elastic body stockings
- Sleeping with head elevated
- Increasing salt intake
- Fludrocortisone to expand fluid volume

Interventions for cardiac denervation and abnormal cardiovascular response to exercise include:
- Avoiding strenuous exercise and straining
- Stress testing prior to initiating a new activity program
- Avoiding hypoglycemia, which can cause arrhythmias

Micro and Macroalbuminuria

Microalbuminuria is defined as the persistent presence of albumin in the urine in the range of 30 – 299 mg/24 hr. It is considered to be the first stage of nephropathy in type 1 diabetes and a marker for nephropathy in type 2 diabetes. Microalbuminuria is also a marker of increased cardiovascular risk and is associated with retinopathy in diabetes.

Macroalbuminuria is defined as albuminuria greater than or equal to 300 mg/24 hr. This greatly increases the risk for progression to end stage renal disease.

Interventions to delay progression of renal disease include:
- Achievement of normal or near-normal glycemia
- Blood pressure control to ≤ 130/80 mmHg
- Use of ACE inhibitors* (or substitute with ARB)
- Stage-based reduction in dietary protein intake
- Additional therapy to lower blood pressure, which may include calcium channel blockers, diuretics and beta blockers

*ACE inhibitors also prevent major cardiovascular events and related mortality in people with diabetes.

Hypertension and Diabetic Nephropathy

Hypertension is considered the most significant factor in accelerating the progression of established renal disease. This is true for both systolic and diastolic pressures.

The American Diabetes Association (ADA) recommends blood pressure ≤ 130/80 mmHg for the prevention of renal complications in patients with diabetes.

Lifestyle modifications to reduce blood pressure include weight loss (if needed), exercise, tobacco cessation, and reduced salt and alcohol intake. If lifestyle modifications do not result in reaching the blood pressure goal, angiotensin-converting enzyme (ACE) inhibitors are considered the first-line pharmacologic intervention. If these medications produce side effects, angiotensin II receptor blockers (ARBs) are substituted. The most common side effect of ACE inhibitors is cough. Angioedema is a less common but more serious adverse effect.

Studies indicate that reduction of blood pressure may reduce the risk for microvascular complications.

Clients with diabetes should self-monitor their blood pressure as a part of comprehensive self-management. Educators should evaluate the client's technique to ensure accurate readings.

Macrovascular Disease

Macrovascular disease comprises both arteriosclerosis and atherosclerosis. It accounts for more morbidity, mortality and cost than any other complication of diabetes.

Arteriosclerosis is a condition in which the walls of arteries and veins become thicker and lose elasticity.

Atherosclerosis describes the process of plaque formation within blood vessel walls, especially the arteries.

Macrovascular disease affects the cerebral, coronary and peripheral vessels, causing 3 types of macrovascular disease in people with diabetes.

They are:
- Coronary artery disease
  o This develops at an earlier age and has a more aggressive course in people with diabetes.
  o Women with diabetes lose their gender protection from atherosclerosis.
  o People with diabetes are more likely to have an adverse outcome from acute coronary events.
- Cerebral vascular disease in people with diabetes results in 3 – 5 times greater risk for death from stroke than in the population without diabetes.
- Peripheral vascular disease in people with diabetes, along with peripheral neuropathy, accounts for approximately 50% of all nontraumatic lower limb amputations in the United States.

Preventing the Onset or Progression of Macrovascular Disease
Management of hypertension in diabetes is aggressive. It often involves initiating antihypertensive medications even if there is only a modest elevation of blood pressure. An angiotensin-converting enzyme (ACE) inhibitor is usually the first drug of choice.

Smoking cessation is of utmost importance due to the adverse effects of smoking on the vascular system. Routine assessment of smoking status and advice to quit when applicable are important.

Dyslipidemia is managed first with lifestyle interventions, such as low-fat diet, exercise and weight loss, if necessary. Statins or other medications to treat dyslipidemia are recommended for most patients with diabetes.

Aspirin therapy helps overcome the hypercoagulability associated with the insulin resistance syndrome. Aspirin is recommended for people with risk factors such as age over 40, smoking, hypertension, albuminuria and dyslipidemia. The usual dose is 81 mg per day, though higher doses are used in cases of higher risk. Clopidogrel may be used as an alternative to aspirin.

Risk for Coronary Artery Disease

People with diabetes who do not have coronary heart disease (CHD) are at similar risk for a coronary event as people without diabetes who have CHD.

Coronary artery disease is responsible for 50 – 60% of all deaths in people with diabetes.

Although female gender normally provides a degree of cardiovascular protection, women with diabetes lose this natural safeguard. Therefore, efforts to reduce macrovascular risk in women with diabetes should be as aggressive as efforts to decrease the risk in men.

Common symptoms of acute coronary insufficiency include:
- Angina
- Anxiety
- Diaphoresis
- Shortness of breath

It is important to remember that a significant number of people with diabetes have atypical myocardial infarction, also known as "silent MI," in which they do not display the normal MI symptoms.

Peripheral Artery Disease

PAD is a vascular disorder involving obstruction of arterial blood flow to vessels outside the coronary and cerebral systems. Up to one-third of people with diabetes over the age of 50 suffer from this condition. Elevated levels of C-reactive protein (CRP) in diabetes are responsible for the inflammation and cellular derangements that lead to PAD.

The presence of PAD serves as a marker for concomitant coronary and cerebral vascular disease. In diabetes, additional risk factors are:
- Duration of diabetes
- African American or Hispanic ethnicity
- Hyperglycemia
- Peripheral neuropathy
- Smoking
- Older age
- Dyslipidemia
- Hyperhomocysteinemia

The most common symptom of PAD is intermittent claudication. This produces cramping in the calves, thighs and buttocks that occurs with activity and is alleviated with rest. The pain is described as a fullness, aching or itching sensation. Clients with these symptoms should be referred for medical examination.

<u>Treatment and Client Education for Peripheral Artery Disease</u>
Interventions for PAD include the same lifestyle modifications recommended cardiovascular disease. These include smoking cessation, hypertension and lipid management, healthy diet, aspirin therapy and glycemic control. Tobacco cessation is especially important as it is associated with increased risk for amputation.

Although intermittent claudication causes pain with walking, clients should be instructed to continue exercising. Walking programs improve intermittent claudication by increasing blood flow to lower extremities and initiating development of collateral circulation.

Clients with PAD need education on prevention of injury to the feet and prompt care of problems since decreased blood flow impedes the healing process. Footwear that fits properly and provides adequate protection is crucial. Clients should learn to perform daily foot inspections and be taught the signs and symptoms of infection or inadequate healing. For those unable to do their own foot inspection, family members or other caregivers should be identified.

Foot Screening

Foot screening identifies the likelihood of lower-extremity complications related to diabetes, such as ulceration and amputation.

History of lower-extremity ulceration, use of insulin and duration of diabetes greater than 10 years are risk factors. Having previous ulceration or amputation automatically places the person at high risk, with no further screening or examination necessary. Deformities such as Charcot foot, hammer toes or claw toes also predict amputation.

Sensory neuropathy is an important risk factor for foot complications. To determine loss of protective sensation, a 5.07 gram monofilament is applied to several spots on the bottom of the foot. Clients should have their eyes closed during this exam. If the monofilament cannot be detected, the client has lost protective sensation and is at risk for undetected injury and subsequent complications.

Loss of vibratory sensation is a predictor of foot ulceration. This is tested using a 128-cycle tuning fork or a biothesiometer at the big toe.

Charcot Foot

Charcot foot is a complication of diabetes related to peripheral and autonomic neuropathy. Repeated trauma to insensitive, neuropathic joints leads to joint destruction and severe deformities of foot structure.

Acute Charcot foot appears unilaterally as a swollen and warm foot, often appearing like an infection without any outward signs of skin breakdown. Inspection may reveal loss of the arch, producing a "rocker bottom" shape to sole.

In spite of the severe injury, many patients do not feel pain due to neuropathic loss of sensation. They may continue to walk on the injured foot, causing further joint destruction.

Immediate referral for orthopedic evaluation is crucial when Charcot foot is detected. Primary treatment involves non-weight-bearing status on the affected foot. Non-weight-bearing casts are often used to stabilize the foot while the healing process is monitored radiologically. Following healing, corrective shoes are needed to accommodate the change in foot shape.

Selection of Footwear

People with diabetes should wear protective footwear at all times, even in their own homes, at the beach and at swimming pools.

Those who have lost protective sensation should have their shoes fitted by a professional. Sensory loss can impair the ability to recognize that shoes are not fitting properly.

Characteristics of a safe, protective shoe include:
- Oxford style or having a wide Velcro strap so that fit can be modified as feet swell later in the day.
- Plenty of room for the toes. Toe box should allow "wiggle room" and be wide enough to accommodate conditions such as wide feet or bunions.
- Made of leather or other breathable material. Avoid plastic or shoes made of "man-made" materials.
- Adequate cushioning and support for the soles of the feet.

Other safety tips include:
- Check inside shoes before putting them on.
- Change shoes and socks during the day if they become moist from sweating or water.
- Wear socks with shoes. Socks should be made from materials that wick moisture away from skin.

Teach Client to Do Self-Foot Exam

Clients with neuropathy should perform a visual and manual self-foot exam daily. Although clients with intact sensation are likely to perceive foot injuries, it is good practice for them to check their feet each day anyway.

The client's visual acuity should be assessed prior to teaching. Those with visual impairment will not be able to perform an adequate visual inspection and will need the help of another person. If necessary, a manual inspection can substitute for a visual inspection. Mirrors and magnifiers can be used when poor mobility prohibits full foot inspection.

The client should be instructed to look at all areas of the feet: tops, bottoms, sides and between toes. They should look for signs of skin breakdown, pressure areas from shoes, blisters, calluses, dry cracks, ingrown toenails and fungal infections such as athlete's foot. Any of these conditions should be monitored and a healthcare provider promptly consulted if there are any signs of infection or failure to resolve.

Routine Foot Care

Wash feet daily with gentle soap and warm water as part of the daily bathing routine. Foot soaks are not recommended. Dry thoroughly between toes to prevent accumulation of moisture, which can lead to fungal growth.

Moisturizing lotion or cream may be applied to dry skin but avoid getting it between the toes. This adds moisture to an area already susceptible to fungal infection. Use unscented, non-alcohol-based lotions. Foot powder may be applied sparingly if the feet tend to sweat.

Nail faces should be filed as needed to keep them smooth and gently contoured to the shape of the toes. The ends of the nails should be cut straight across, avoiding sharp angles at the corners, which can cause ingrown toenails. Since nails are softer after bathing, this is a good time to perform nail care, especially if nails are thick or hard. Clients with sensory neuropathy, peripheral vascular disease or a history of foot ulcer should have a healthcare provider cut their toenails.

Progression of Foot Injury

The most common cause of foot ulcers is minor repetitive trauma, such as walking on a bony prominence or repeated pressure from shoes that are too tight.

Many minor traumas are preventable and come from poorly fitting shoes, walking barefoot, foreign objects in the shoes or inappropriate treatment of corns, calluses or blisters. Most amputations are preventable with client education about footwear, foot inspection and proper care of common problems.

Ulceration involves full-thickness skin trauma that infiltrates the subcutaneous tissue. Proper wound management is essential to prevent infection and amputation. Management of foot ulceration includes optimization of glycemic control, debridement as needed, applying dressings and protection from further trauma to allow healing.

Signs of infection include redness, swelling, warm, continuous drainage and failure to heal. Localized infection of 30 days duration or less can usually be effectively treated with oral antibiotics. Clients with signs of systemic infection, such as severe hyperglycemia or fever, require prompt emergency referral.

Honeymoon Period

The honeymoon period is a remission phase that occurs early in the natural course of type 1 diabetes. It is characterized by a temporary improvement in endogenous insulin secretion and a decreased need for injected insulin.

The temporary increase in endogenous insulin production is due to decreased inflammation of the Islets of Langerhans caused by the original autoimmune assault. When exogenous insulin is started, inflammation of the beta cells subsides and the beta cells resume insulin production. As the autoimmune disease progresses, these revived cells eventually lose their function and the need for injected insulin resumes or increases.

The honeymoon period typically lasts between 3 and 12 months and is more common in young adults with type 1 diabetes than in younger children with the disease.

During the honeymoon period, insulin doses are decreased to prevent hypoglycemia.

Clients should be prepared for the honeymoon period so that they do not question the diagnosis of type 1 diabetes. If necessary, they should be supported emotionally as the need for insulin inevitably increases.

Dawn Phenomenon

The dawn phenomenon refers to normal hormonal fluctuations that trigger the liver to release excessive glucose in the latter part of the nightly sleep cycle. It is often responsible for elevated fasting glucose levels in the person with diabetes.

People who do not have diabetes produce the additional insulin needed to maintain normal glucose levels at this time. People with type 2 diabetes often see higher blood glucose results in the morning due to the dawn phenomenon. Metformin can be an effective medication to address the dawn phenomenon because it decreases glucose production by the liver.

People who require endogenous insulin need to adjust the dose and timing of their medication to provide for a greater insulin need during the pre-waking hours. Long-acting insulin and insulin pump therapy are especially helpful in regulating the variable blood glucose pattern produced by the dawn phenomenon.

People who work rotating shifts or suffer from jet lag require careful adjustment of insulin therapy to accommodate the dawn phenomenon.

Somogyi Phenomenon

The existence of the Somogyi phenomenon is controversial. However, some people believe it may be a rare cause of fasting hyperglycemia. Theoretically, the Somogyi phenomenon is a rebound effect of nocturnal hypoglycemia. As the blood glucose level drops during prolonged fasting, the counter-regulatory hormones cause an excess release of glucose from the liver as a compensatory mechanism.

Continuous glucose monitoring (CGM) can detect if this phenomenon is causing morning hyperglycemia. Alternatively, sometimes patients are asked to awaken during the night to check their blood glucose to determine if hypoglycemia is triggering the Somogyi effect. This is often not practical as it is difficult to determine the precise time to awaken for the test.

Basal insulin, such as NPH or glargine, usually affects the morning blood glucose. Regardless of the cause of early morning hyperglycemia, adjustment of these insulins is often indicated to offset the rise in blood glucose.

Hypoglycemic Unawareness

Normally, low blood glucose triggers the release of counter-regulatory hormones, such as glucagon and epinephrine. Among other things, these hormones are responsible for producing the physical symptoms of hypoglycemia, such as palpitations, sweating and anxiety.

In hypoglycemic unawareness, however, the body fails to release or only produces a small amount of counter-regulatory hormones. As a result, the hypoglycemic patient may experience no symptoms and remain unaware that he or she needs to take action to prevent subsequent coma. Or, symptoms of hypoglycemia may occur at much lower glucose levels than usual, substantially decreasing the window of opportunity for prompt action. Hypoglycemic unawareness clearly presents a serious safety issue, especially for patients with diabetes who require insulin.

In the past, autonomic neuropathy was believed to be the sole cause of hypoglycemic unawareness. However, recent findings suggest that it is largely due to a lack of adaptation by the body to previous episodes of hypoglycemia. Longer duration of diabetes and a history of frequent hypoglycemic episodes increase the risk for this condition.

Management and Education Considerations for Hypoglycemic Unawareness
Hypoglycemic unawareness refers to the loss of normal counter-regulatory action in response to low blood glucose. The resulting safety issues present a management challenge, especially for people who require insulin.

The first step in management is usually liberalization of glycemic goals to prevent hypoglycemia. For the patient with hypoglycemic unawareness on a basal bolus insulin regimen, greater use of long-acting insulin and smaller boluses are recommended.

Although longer duration of diabetes increases the risk for developing hypoglycemic unawareness, repeated episodes of hypoglycemia increase the risk further. To delay the onset of this condition, care should be taken to prevent hypoglycemia in the earlier stages of diabetes treatment. This presents a challenge and a barrier to optimizing glycemic control.

In some cases, the normal counter-regulatory response can be restored with treatment programs to prevent hypoglycemia, especially in those who do not have autonomic neuropathy.

Clients with hypoglycemic unawareness and their significant others require education about careful insulin dosing, increased home glucose monitoring, caution while driving and wearing diabetes medical identification.

Sick Day Management of Child with Type 1 Diabetes

Illness in the child with type 1 diabetes presents significant risk for diabetic ketoacidosis (DKA). Colds, flu and other infections can cause hyperglycemia. In infants, hyperglycemia can also be caused by teething or following routine immunizations.

The primary goal of sick day management is to maintain hydration and prevent severe hyperglycemia. Consistent oral hydration with $\frac{1}{2}$ – 1 cup of sugar-free fluid every hour is needed.

Urine ketone testing is used to monitor sick day response. Urine ketones should be checked when blood glucose is 300 mg/dl or greater. The presence of moderate to large amounts of ketones requires additional insulin. If the child is not eating, fluids that contain sugar should be given. If hypoglycemia occurs, a glucagon injection may be needed.

Parents and caregivers should know that DKA is a medical emergency and should seek immediate medical care for the following:
- Prolonged vomiting or diarrhea
- Not taking fluids
- Lethargy
- Rapid deep breathing
- Persistent hyperglycemia and /or ketonuria

Managing Diabetes during Sick Days

The physical stress of illness can trigger a counter-regulatory response resulting in hyperglycemia. This is especially common with colds, flu and other types of infection. Being ill is a risk factor for the hyperglycemic emergencies of hyperosmolar hyperglycemic state (HHS) and diabetic ketoacidosis (DKA). Both of these conditions can produce profound dehydration and electrolyte imbalance.

Management guidelines for sick days include:
- Continue to take oral diabetes medication and insulin, even if not eating normally.
- Stop taking metformin if dehydrated and contact physician.
- Follow regular meal plan if able. Supplement with a cup of non-caloric fluid every hour.
- If unable to eat, drink $\frac{1}{2}$ – one cup sugar-containing fluid every hour.
- Check blood glucose every 2 – 4 hours while awake.
- Notify healthcare provider for:
  - Persistent vomiting or diarrhea
  - Blood glucose consistently over 300 mg/dl
  - Temperature greater than 101°F
  - Small or greater amounts of ketones in the urine

Insulin Pump during Surgery

For patients using a continuous subcutaneous insulin infusion (CSII) device, also known as an insulin pump, options for surgery and the postoperative period should be discussed with the surgeon and anesthesiologist. If the device is to be used during surgery, the anesthesiologist must demonstrate an acceptable level of comfort with managing it.

When an insulin pump is to be in place during surgery, the catheter should be inserted at a site away from the surgical field and reinforced with extra tape. A new catheter should be inserted 12 – 24 hours before the surgery to ensure adequate insulin infusion.

If hospital policy allows, patients who are alert and oriented should be allowed to manage their own insulin pump therapy, assuming they have managed well prior to hospitalization.

If the pump is to be discontinued, intravenous or subcutaneous insulin should be given prior to discontinuation.

Physiologic Effects of Illness and Surgery

Physiological stressors such as illness, infection, surgery and trauma can disrupt normal metabolic homeostasis. Counter-regulatory hormone secretion is increased during these times and has the following effects on blood glucose:
- Stimulates the release of glucose from the liver
- Inhibits the action of insulin
- Inhibits the uptake of glucose by the muscle
- Diverts blood from the periphery, possibly affecting the absorption of injected insulin

The subsequent hyperglycemia causes osmotic diuresis and can lead to dehydration and loss of sodium, potassium, phosphorus and magnesium.

In type 1 diabetes, insufficient insulin and inadequate carbohydrate intake can cause lipolysis and ketogenesis. If ketosis is not treated, diabetic ketoacidosis (DKA) can result.

In type 2 diabetes, significant ketosis usually does not develop because endogenous insulin secretion continues. However, severe hyperglycemia, profound dehydration and electrolyte imbalance can result in these clients.

Hyperglycemia and Hypoglycemia in Surgical Patient

Because it adversely affects white blood cell function, hyperglycemia is associated with impaired wound healing and increased risk for infection. It also increases platelet aggregation and makes red blood cells more rigid, resulting in decreased circulation through the small vessels. Additionally, high blood glucose interferes with normal protein synthesis, which is essential for healing the surgical wound. For optimal healing, blood glucose should remain at 200 mg/dl or less in the postoperative patient.

Elevated blood glucose increases the risk for ketoacidosis, especially in the patient with type 1 diabetes. Even moderate hyperglycemia can induce ketosis in type 1 patients who are undergoing surgery.

Hyperglycemia significantly increases the risk for electrolyte imbalance and fluid volume depletion in surgical patients with diabetes.

During the operative and the immediate postoperative periods, surgical patients are unable to detect and report symptoms of hypoglycemia, placing them at risk for coma. For this reason, frequent monitoring of blood glucose is required for all anesthetized patients with diabetes.

Implications for Type 1 Diabetes Having Surgery

Preoperative patients with type 1 diabetes should have surgery scheduled for early in the morning to prevent prolonged fasting. If this is not possible, intravenous therapy for those who are not allowed to eat is required to maintain homeostasis. These infusions may include insulin, glucose solution and electrolytes as needed.

A diabetologist or endocrinologist is usually consulted about intraoperative insulin and fluid management of the surgical patient with type 1 diabetes. Protocols for insulin administration during surgery are used.

People who use an insulin pump may leave the pump attached with a basal rate running during surgery. Supplemental short or rapid-acting insulin is given intravenously as needed.

Frequent blood glucose and ketone monitoring are necessary for these patients. During the operative period, blood glucose is monitored every $\frac{1}{2}$ – 1hour and urine ketones are checked every 4 – 6 hours.

Subcutaneous insulin must be given 30 minutes prior to discontinuing the intravenous insulin infusion.

Patient Education for Type 2 Diabetes Having Surgery

Medications:
- Follow instructions given by the doctor for taking diabetes medication the day of surgery. Sometimes the oral medications are allowed the morning of surgery and sometimes they are stopped the evening before.
- Chlorpropamide, a longer-acting sulfonylurea, is normally discontinued 48 – 72 hours before surgery.
- Metformin is usually discontinued the morning of surgery. Instruct the patient not to resume metformin postoperatively until they are eating and drinking normally and urinating sufficiently.
- Many patients with type 2 diabetes who normally use oral diabetes medications need insulin during the perioperative and postoperative periods. Assure patients that this is due to the physiologic stress of illness and surgery and that preventing hyperglycemia promotes healing. Reassure the patient that most people are able to resume their regular medication regimens postoperatively.

Patients should be aware that dextrose is commonly used for people with diabetes having surgery. This can prevent them from thinking there is a mistake in receiving a fluid with sugar.

Traveling with Diabetes

People with diabetes should carry medications, insulin, syringes and testing supplies in their carry-on luggage when traveling by air. Medications and supplies should be protected from temperature extremes.

People at risk need to carry fast-acting carbohydrate to treat hypoglycemia. To prepare for long flights, delays and cancelled flights, they should also carry a meal. A travel companion should know the signs, symptoms and treatment of hypoglycemia. Clients should wear medical identification stating that they have diabetes.

The following guidelines are used for making insulin adjustments when traveling across time zones:
- If the time change is 3 or fewer hours, adjust timing of insulin injections by one-half hour ahead or back, depending upon the direction of travel, until resumption of normal schedule.
- If traveling eastbound overseas, reduce basal insulin on the day of travel since it will be a shorter day. Maintain the same bolus regimen.
- If traveling westbound overseas, add injections of short-acting insulin every 4 – 6 hours, before meals, to compensate for the longer day.

Nutritional Considerations for Older Adult

Elderly clients with diabetes have a higher risk for failure to thrive and malnutrition than younger adult clients. Glycemic goals should take into account risk factors that can have a negative impact on nutritional status in this age group. These include:
- Decreased energy needs
- Decreased physical function that impairs ability to shop and cook
- Depression
- Cognitive impairment
- Financial constraints
- Poor dentition or tooth loss
- Altered nutrient absorption
- Decreased thirst sensation
- Social isolation

For frail elderly residents with diabetes in nursing facilities, providing adequate nutrition is the primary concern. Glycemic control is best addressed by implementing a meal plan that provides a consistent amount of carbohydrate from day to day. Specific calorie goals, special "diabetic diets" or "no concentrated sweets" diets are no longer considered appropriate for this population.

Medication Considerations for Older Adult

Elderly patients with diabetes are sometimes treated with sulfonylureas. Glipizide is often preferred over glyburide because it is shorter acting and has fewer hepatic metabolites. First-generation sulfonylureas, such as tolazamide, are rarely used in this population because of their long half-life. The risk for hypoglycemia should always be considered in the elderly because they are more likely to have hypoglycemic unawareness.

Metformin use is restricted in many geriatric patients due to renal or hepatic insufficiency.

Use of thiazolidinediones in the elderly has not been widely studied.

Medication regimens should be simplified as much as possible since polypharmacy is a common problem in the older adult population.

Cost of medication may be an issue for seniors with limited income.

The need for insulin to control blood glucose increases with age due to the progressive nature of diabetes. Teaching should be adapted for alterations in function, such as vision loss and arthritis, as well as the slower mental processing that is a normal change with aging.

Hypoglycemia in the Elderly

Elderly people with diabetes have a higher risk for hypoglycemia, are more at risk for hypoglycemic unawareness and are more likely to confuse hypoglycemia with other disease symptoms.

There are numerous reasons why this population has a higher risk for hypoglycemia. Decreased renal function can alter the clearance of medications that lower blood glucose while the counter-regulatory response to hypoglycemia is blunted. Polypharmacy, inadequate or erratic food intake and slowed intestinal absorption are additional risk factors.

The elderly and their significant others should learn about the signs and symptoms of hypoglycemia and be cautioned to not confuse these with other disease symptoms, the side effects of medications or normal aging.

Glycemic goals for the elderly are sometimes liberalized to avoid hypoglycemic episodes. Oral agents that do not produce hypoglycemic effects may be preferred for these patients.

Older adults at risk for hypoglycemia may need emergency systems in place, such as an emergency pager. They should wear medical identification stating that they have diabetes.

Pregnancy

Preconception Care
All women of childbearing age should be tested for diabetes prior to conception if they have risk factors for diabetes.

Starting at puberty, all women of childbearing age with diabetes should be counseled about the potential risks of unplanned pregnancy. Family planning resources should be offered. The importance of preconception care should be incorporated into all routine medical visits for appropriate patients.

For women with pre-existing diabetes, A1C levels should be 7.0% or less before conception is attempted. Glycemic control prior to conception and in early pregnancy reduces the risk of birth defects to a level similar to that of the general population.

A preconception workup includes evaluation and treatment, if indicated, for diabetic retinopathy, nephropathy, neuropathy and cardiovascular disease.

Medication assessment is also important for such patients since many drugs used for the treatment of diabetes are contraindicated or not advised in pregnancy. These include statins, ACE inhibitors and most oral antidiabetic agents.

Fetal and Neonatal Complications Associated with Maternal Hyperglycemia
Perinatal complications can be correlated with the level of maternal glycemic control during pregnancy.

Planned pregnancy is of critical importance in women with diabetes because fetal organ formation takes place in the first 8 weeks of gestation, at which time many women are unaware that they are pregnant. Uncontrolled blood glucose in the first trimester of pregnancy is associated with spontaneous abortion and congenital malformations, such as neural tube defects, heart anomalies and renal anomalies.

The placenta becomes fully grown and functioning by about 18 weeks gestation at which time the fetus can develop metabolic complications secondary to maternal hyperglycemia. These complications include macrosomia,* increased risk for childhood obesity and glucose intolerance, stillbirth, respiratory distress syndrome and hyperbilirubinemia.

Hypoglycemia in the neonate is the most common complication of second and third trimester hyperglycemia in the mother. Neonatal hypoglycemia is defined as:

- 35 mg/dl in full-term infants
- 25 mg/dl or less in preterm infants

Macrosomia is abnormally high birth weight.

Maternal Complications Related to Diabetes
Maternal complications of uncontrolled blood glucose during pregnancy include hypertension, preterm labor and delivery, cesarean section and pyelonephritis.

Hypertension in such women may include pregnancy-induced hypertension (preeclampsia) and chronic hypertension. For chronic hypertension, the usual antihypertensive medications, such as ACE inhibitors and ARBs, are contraindicated during pregnancy.

Calcium channel blockers and labetalol are often substituted. Target blood pressure during pregnancy is 110/65 – 129/79 mm Hg.

Hypertension, whether pregnancy-induced or preexisting, is the most significant risk factor for progression of retinopathy in pregnancy.

Women with preexisting early renal disease should be encouraged to attempt pregnancy as early as feasible because pregnancy presents a risk for worsening renal impairment in these patients.

While diabetes is not an absolute indication for cesarean, the risk is increased in this population.

Women with proliferative retinopathy often require cesarean delivery to avoid the Valsalva maneuver, which could cause retinal hemorrhage. High birth weight neonates are at increased risk of shoulder dystocia from vaginal delivery, necessitating cesarean delivery in some cases.

Psychosocial Issues When Educating Clients about Diabetes and Pregnancy
Having diabetes does not appear to affect fertility.

The chance of having a child with type 1 diabetes when the mother has type 1 diabetes is 2%. For the child having a father with type 1 diabetes, the risk is 6%.

Glycemic control during pregnancy is correlated with the risk for spontaneous abortion (SA). When the patient has good blood glucose control during pregnancy, the risk for SA is about the same as for the general population.

The risk for congenital birth defects is greatly increased when the mother has markedly elevated A1C levels during pregnancy. Maternal serum alpha-fetoprotein screening can detect neural tube defects. Ultrasonography can detect anomalies of the central nervous system, heart and kidneys. Patients should be made aware that these tests are not 100% sensitive for detecting these problems.

Those planning pregnancy should consider the possible financial challenges associated with a complicated pregnancy. This may include increased surveillance requiring more medical tests and appointments. The potential need for more missed work days should be taken into consideration.

Diabetic Retinopathy during Pregnancy
Certain placental hormones cause vascular changes that can accelerate retinopathy.

Women of childbearing age with retinopathy should be educated about the effect that pregnancy can have on their eyes. Preconception planning for women with diabetes should include a thorough ophthalmologic exam.

Nonproliferative retinopathy is not a contraindication for pregnancy. While there is significant risk that nonproliferative retinopathy will progress during pregnancy, this is expected to reverse after delivery.

Results of studies are mixed concerning the risk for the progression of proliferative retinopathy in pregnant women whose eyes have been stabilized with photocoagulation prior to pregnancy.

Those with untreated proliferative retinopathy have the highest risk for progression during pregnancy. Pregnancy in these women is contraindicated until their eyes can be stabilized with photocoagulation.

Many women with proliferative retinopathy deliver their babies by cesarean section or vacuum extracted vaginal delivery to avoid pushing during childbirth.

Gestational Diabetes
Gestational diabetes (GDM) is broadly defined as a condition of carbohydrate intolerance at the onset or first recognition of pregnancy. This definition includes women with existing but undiagnosed diabetes prior to pregnancy. In the United States, it is estimated that about 2% of women of childbearing age have undiagnosed diabetes.

In 2009, new criteria for the diagnosis of GDM were established. The current method for screening and diagnosis of GDM is:
- Screen all women for diabetes risk at first prenatal visit.
- Test between 24 – 28 weeks gestation in all pregnant women of average risk.*
- Use 75-gram oral glucose tolerance test (OGTT); 50-gram test is no longer used.
- Diagnose GDM when:
  - Fasting blood glucose is ≥ 92 mg/dl
  - 1-hour post-OGTT result is ≥ 180 mg/dl
  - 2-hour post-OGTT result is ≥ 158 mg/dl
- Only 1 of the abnormal values listed above is required for diagnosis.

*Women with high risk for diabetes should be tested for GDM as soon as possible. If first test is negative, retest again at 24 – 28 weeks gestation. Risk factors include:
- History of GDM
- Family history of diabetes
- Obesity
- Glycosuria

How Pregnancy Affects Normal Metabolism
Normal pregnancy is a diabetogenic state. Hormones produced during pregnancy, such as progesterone, human placental hormone and prolactin, lead to an insulin-resistant state. Normally, blood insulin levels double or triple during the third trimester due to increased needs of the

placenta. For women with pre-existing insulin resistance or gestational diabetes, the relative amount of available insulin remains insufficient.

In pregnancy, the glycemic response to food consumption results in greater and more prolonged elevation in blood glucose.

During the second and third trimesters of pregnancy, the risk for maternal ketosis increases. This should be avoided since ketones have an adverse affect on the fetus. Education includes advising the client to refrain from fasting and unsupervised weight loss and to check for urine ketones in the later stages of pregnancy.

In the immediate postpartum period, insulin sensitivity increases due to the sudden drop in placental hormones and most women promptly return to their pre-pregnancy insulin requirements.

Treatment Goals for Gestational Diabetes
Regular self-monitoring of blood glucose is highly recommended for all women with GDM. Plasma glucose targets are as follows:
- Premeal, bedtime, and overnight glucose: 60-99 mg/dl
- Peak postprandial glucose: 100-129 mg/dl

Medical nutrition therapy (MNT), following a carbohydrate-controlled meal plan, is the initial focus of treatment. Because early glycemic control is important, prompt intervention by a registered dietitian is recommended. The goals of MNT are normoglycemia, adequate nutrition, appropriate weight gain and absence of ketosis. For obese women with GDM, weight loss is controversial. If attempted, it must be medically supervised and caution must be taken to prevent ketosis.

Unless contraindicated, exercise is recommended to improve glucose tolerance and potentially prevent the need for insulin injections.

When diet and exercise do not produce desired results, insulin is the most commonly used medication to treat GDM. Glyburide and metformin have also been studied and may be used in some cases of GDM.

Postpartum Considerations for Gestational Diabetes
Most women with GDM return to normal blood glucose levels shortly after delivery, although 40 – 60% will develop type 2 diabetes within 10 years. Client education and medical surveillance are indicated for the prevention and early detection of subsequent type 2 diabetes in women with GDM.

Following childbirth, the patient should continue self-monitoring of blood glucose until normoglycemia is reached. A 75-gram oral glucose tolerance test is indicated at approximately 6 weeks postpartum.

Women with a history of GDM should have a fasting plasma glucose test every year and a 75-gram oral glucose tolerance test every 3 years to screen for type 2 diabetes. They should be educated to request these screening tests if they change health-care providers.

Education includes the importance of a healthy diet and BMI, using the USDA dietary guidelines, and regular exercise (after medical clearance has been obtained). Since many clients with GDM are overweight or obese, initial weight loss to below 5 – 7% of preconception weight is indicated for the prevention of type 2 diabetes.

Breastfeeding for the Woman with Diabetes

Many women mistakenly believe that they cannot breastfeed if they have diabetes, whether chronic or gestational. Education includes informing these clients that breastfeeding is not contraindicated but is, in fact, highly recommended. Perceived barriers to breastfeeding should be explored.

Breastfeeding has many advantages for women with previous gestational diabetes (GDM) and should be strongly encouraged in this group. Breastfeeding lowers glucose levels postpartum and reduces the risk for future development of type 2 diabetes. It also mobilizes fat stores and promotes weight loss, which is important for the 50% of GDM patients who are obese.

For women with pre-existing diabetes who use insulin, breastfeeding may enable the insulin dosage to be reduced. These women should self-monitor blood glucose frequently and be aware of the increased risk for hypoglycemia. Sometimes, taking a snack before breastfeeding and an overall increase in daily calorie consumption are recommended.

Ketone Monitoring during Pregnancy

During pregnancy, the blood glucose value at which women can spill ketones is lower, placing them at greater risk for diabetic ketoacidosis (DKA). In rare cases, ketoacidosis occurs in pregnant women with normal blood glucose levels.

The elevated risk for ketosis is caused by increased fat catabolism during pregnancy. Ketones cross the placenta and can pose a risk to the fetus. Fetal exposure to ketones is associated with fetal demise and lower IQ scores.

Routine monitoring of urine and/or blood ketones is necessary during pregnancy; urine ketones are monitored with the first morning specimen. Indications for additional ketone testing are blood glucose $\geq$ 200 mg/dl, significant vomiting with morning sickness or other illness. The most common cause of ketosis is infection.

When ketones are present with normal or low blood glucose, inadequate food intake is suspected. When ketones are concurrent with elevated glucose, ketosis is imminent.

Nutritional Considerations for the Pregnant Woman

The general goals of nutrition therapy during pregnancy are to provide sufficient nutrition for mother and fetus, to promote appropriate fetal growth and maternal weight gain and to maintain glycemic control.

Nutrients of particular concern during pregnancy include protein, calcium, iron and folate.

Recommendations for weight gain depend upon the preconception weight status of the mother. Obese women are generally recommended to gain only as much as the products of conception, approximately 15 pounds. Weight loss for these women is occasionally recommended but is controversial.

Women of healthy weight are recommended to gain 1 pound per week during the 2nd and 3rd trimester. Overweight women should gain only $\frac{1}{2}$ pound per week during the last 2 trimesters.

Consistency of the timing and amount of food intake is especially important for pregnant women using insulin. Bedtime snacks are often needed to prevent ketosis related to overnight starvation.

Non-nutritive sweeteners, such as aspartame and acesulfame K, are considered safe for use during pregnancy.

<u>Morning Sickness</u>
Any time a pregnant woman is unable to eat or keep food down, there is a risk for the development of ketosis. Careful monitoring of urine and/or blood ketones is recommended when a client has significant morning sickness.

Hypoglycemia can produce morning sickness. Women at risk should be instructed to check blood glucose when nausea appears and to treat low blood glucose promptly and appropriately.

Vomiting presents a challenge for clients who use insulin. If vomiting occurs after taking the short-acting pre-meal insulin, the client should take enough glucagon to raise the blood glucose 30 – 40 mg/dl to prevent hypoglycemia. The glucagon is effective for 1 – 2 hours, during which time morning sickness may subside and food can be taken. If the client remains unable to eat and blood glucose declines, additional glucagon is needed until the peak action of the insulin has abated. Clients should contact their healthcare provider if they develop persistent nausea and vomiting.

Celiac Disease in Type 1 Diabetes

Celiac disease associated with type 1 diabetes is often overlooked. Its prevalence rate is approximately 4 – 6% among people with type 1 diabetes.

Celiac disease is an autoimmune disorder of the small intestine most commonly seen in people of European descent. It is thought to be triggered by a viral immune response in people with a genetic predisposition.

Celiac disease causes an inability to digest certain nutrients and results in chronic diarrhea, failure to thrive, and loss of energy. A gluten-free diet relieves symptoms and improves general health. This diet must be maintained for life.

People with type 1 diabetes and celiac disease must avoid all wheat-based foods. This can be challenging because gluten is used as an additive in many food products and is found in processed cheese, ground spices, cosmetics, lip balms and even postage stamps.

Examples of grain products appropriate for a gluten-free diet are corn, rice, potatoes and soy.

Clients with celiac disease should be referred to a registered dietitian who can provide education and emotional support for making these complicated dietary adaptations.

Exercise Considerations for the Obese

The majority of obese persons lead sedentary lifestyles. The initial goal is usually to simply increase activity.

The client should be assisted in identifying and overcoming barriers to physical activity. If the client is embarrassed by his or her lack of fitness, solitary exercise or finding a group of people with similar status can be suggested.

Continuous aerobic activity has the most beneficial effect on weight loss and fat burning. A progressive walking program is suitable for many obese clients. Water exercise is a good option for those with joint or foot pain. However, swimming is less likely to produce aerobic effects and weight loss. Obese clients should avoid high-impact exercises that place too much stress on the joints, such as jogging or high-impact aerobics.

Exercise intensity should start at the lower end of the target heart range. Frequency of exercise should be 3 – 5 times per week.

Thyroid Disorders

Thyroid disorders are more common in people with diabetes than the general population.

Since type 1 diabetes is an autoimmune disorder affecting the pancreas, other organs can be affected by the destructive process, including the thyroid. Thyroid dysfunction appears to be more common in people with type 2 diabetes as well.

The most common type of thyroid dysfunction is hypothyroidism. In the person with diabetes, this can affect glucose control and can affect response to medication. When the thyroid level is low, metabolism slows and the action of medications may be prolonged. This can increase the risk for hypoglycemia in clients at risk. Medication doses usually need to be reduced when hypothyroidism presents concurrently with diabetes.

Hyperthyroidism usually causes a worsening of glycemic control and an increased need for insulin. Some of the symptoms of hyperthyroidism, such as rapid or pounding heartbeat, sweating and tremors, can mimic hypoglycemia.

Clients with diabetes should be screened for thyroid disease, even in the absence of symptoms as many cases are subclinical.

Diabetic Foot Ulcers

Diabetic foot wounds are often treated inadequately because patients and healthcare providers do not appreciate the seriousness of a non-healing ulcer. Because underlying osteomyelitis can occur with little evidence of inflammation, treatment may be deferred. Prompt and appropriate treatment of foot ulcers can lead to significant decrease in amputations.

Wound debridement is essential to the treatment of a foot ulcer because it helps move the wound past the inflammatory phase, allowing healing to commence. Debridement involves chemically or mechanically removing necrotic, callused and any other physiologically impaired tissue.

"Offloading" is an ulcer management strategy that requires the patient not to place any weight on the affected foot. Noncompliance rates with this recommendation are high and present a significant barrier to healing. Some healthcare providers have the patient wear a non-removable cast to enforce offloading of the wound.

Meticulous documentation is needed to track the progression of wound healing. This includes objective measurements of wound size and measures of glycemic control.

Yeast and Fungal Infections

Poor glycemic control increases the risk for developing yeast and fungal infection of the skin and nails.

Tinea pedis, also known as athlete's foot, is a common problem in people with diabetes. Avoiding prolonged exposure of the feet to moisture is an important preventive measure. Instruct the client to dry well between the toes after bathing and to avoid wearing moist shoes and socks. Antifungal foot powder can be applied sparingly in the shoes. It is a good idea to alternate shoes from day to day to allow thorough drying in between wearing.

Yeast infections commonly occur in the folds of the skin where moisture can accumulate. Vaginal yeast infections can also occur. Over-the-counter (OTC) products for treating vaginal yeast infections are available. However, a client should only use one if she is having symptoms similar to an episode previously diagnosed by a healthcare professional. These OTC products should not be used more than 4 times per year without medical supervision.

Adaptive Equipment for the Visually Impaired

For measuring insulin, syringe magnifiers may be adequate for many clients with poor vision. Others may benefit from using preset dose gauges that assist with measuring insulin. Other devices measure insulin units by a series of audible or perceptible clicks. Some devices require set up assistance by a person with unimpaired vision.

Insulin pens are prefilled and can be operated non-visually by many people. Although this is not specifically endorsed by the pen manufacturers, many people feel it is a safe practice for appropriate clients.

Some types of insulin pumps have auditory cues and are sometimes appropriate for a visually impaired person. Proper assessment should determine the safety of this for the individual.

For monitoring blood glucose, talking meters are available and regular meters can often be adapted to provide this feature. Some meters have test strips with distinctive tactile features that can assist the user. Blood drop guides are also available to help with placing the blood drop on the test strip.

Sleep Apnea

As many as 50% of people with type 2 diabetes also have sleep apnea. Sleep apnea worsens insulin resistance and increases the risk for cardiovascular events, hypertension and erectile dysfunction.

Symptoms of sleep apnea include:
- Snoring, especially if loudly and frequently
- Breathing cessation or gasping to regain breath while asleep
- Frequent awakening during the night
- Being sleepy during the day
- Having trouble concentrating

Primary prevention of sleep apnea is to achieve and maintain a healthy BMI. Self-treatment options include avoiding alcohol and sleeping on the back. Dental appliances that position the mandible to maintain an open airway are also available. The most effective treatment is the continuous positive air pressure (CPAP) machine.

All patients with diabetes should be routinely screened for sleep apnea. If sleep apnea is suspected, diagnosis can be confirmed with sleep lab studies.

Program Development and Administration

Quantitative and Qualitative Research

Quantitative research translates data into numbers for statistical analysis. It seeks to explain cause-and-effect relationships. Quantitative studies are classified according to the level of control applied and the likelihood that the findings occurred by chance. Grade 1 research evidence implies that the study used a highly controlled and randomized design. Grade 5 means that the evidence is based on a descriptive study or expert opinion.

Qualitative research uses the subject's own words or the researcher's narrative summary of an observed phenomenon. An example of a qualitative study would be to investigate the concept of "becoming diabetic" by analyzing interviews and journals on the subject and extracting common themes.

Both types of research should be conducted with rigorous methods such as attention to detail and strict accuracy. When both types of research are blended to collect data, it is referred to as multi-method research.

Scientific Method

Research is a systematic process that utilizes the scientific method to answer questions. Research findings generate new knowledge and guide clinical practice.

Rigor in research refers to a method that moves in an orderly fashion, applies scrupulous attention to detail and imposes control on the research situation to maximize validity. Research evidence is collected in such a way that it can be reviewed and replicated by others.

The first step of the scientific method is to devise research objectives, questions and hypotheses. The subsequent tasks of the scientific method are to collect and analyze data and report results.

Although rigorous, the process of scientific research is considered flexible and circular. As the study progresses, researchers often have to rework a problem several times. This may be due to new findings from other research or identifying a problem with the initial research design.

Major Studies on Diabetes Glycemic Control

The Diabetes Control and Complications Trial (DCCT) demonstrated a 60% reduction in the development of microvascular complications in intensely-treated people with type 1 diabetes. Over 6.5 years, the mean A1C of the intensive treatment group was 7%, compared to about 9% in the standard treatment group.

The United Kingdom Prospective Diabetes Study (UKPDS) followed newly diagnosed people with type 2 diabetes for 10 years. With intensive glycemic control, yielding a median A1C of 7%, the risk for microvascular complications was significantly reduced. UKDPS also suggested that intensive control can reduce the incidence of heart attack and stroke in type 2 diabetics.

The Action to Control Cardiovascular Risk in Diabetes (ACCORD) study compared the effects of intensive glycemic control on cardiovascular outcomes in people with type 2 diabetes. One arm of this study terminated early due to findings that intensive glycemic control (A1C goal < 6%) was associated with increased mortality of participants. The potential explanations for this are still being studied. Other arms of ACCORD, studying lipid and blood pressure control, continue.

Interpret Blood Glucose Results

Interpretation of food records, medication practices and exercise logs are valuable in interpreting blood glucose values and directing changes in therapy. Medication changes should be made based on blood glucose trends rather than a single reading.

When blood glucose is high after meals, possible causes are:
- too much carbohydrate at the meal
- not enough pre-meal insulin
- inadequate dose of oral agent (except metformin)
- not enough exercise in preceding hours or days

When fasting blood glucose is high, possible causes are:
- not enough basal insulin
- inadequate oral medication in evening or at bedtime

When blood glucose is high most of the time, possible reasons are:
- insufficient medication dose
- patient requires combination therapy
- medication has not been taken for long enough time
- not enough exercise
- too much carbohydrate overall
- excessive stress

When blood glucose values are erratic, possible causes are:
- inconsistent timing of meals or quantity of carbohydrate intake
- irregular insulin injection technique, such as changing injection site from the abdomen to the arm
- insulin has lost potency
- excessive stress

Evaluation

Evaluating Achievement of Educational Objectives
Surveys are easy to design and use. Questions can be given in written or oral form. A disadvantage of surveys is that respondents can interpret questions differently, affecting the reliability of data. Telephone and face-to-face surveys often yield a high response rate.

Chart audits can produce objective data such as laboratory results and adherence to recommendations for preventive services. Chart audits involve reviewing records to capture associations between education and outcomes. Disadvantages of this method are the time required to go through records and the variability of different reviewers' skill in collecting data.

Checklists gather concurrent information and can reveal behavior change and implementation of tasks. Reliability of collected data depends upon the consistency and skill of those collecting the data.

Other methods of evaluation include asking participants to take pre- and post-tests or perform return demonstration of skills taught.

Evaluating a Client's Progress toward Behavioral Goals
Evaluation of client progress toward behavioral goals should be done in a nonjudgmental manner. Intensive diabetes management is rigorous and even those who are adherent may occasionally relax their standards, such as during times of stress or on holidays and vacations. These relapses are expected and do not signify a failure on the part of the client.

The educator can support the client through a relapse by helping identify the cause of the relapse and exploring optimal ways of dealing with it. The client should be supported and encouraged to resume working toward his or her behavioral goals as soon as feasible.

Lifestyle behaviors, such as diet and exercise, can be difficult to maintain for long periods. Therefore, ongoing monitoring and evaluation of these behaviors is indicated. When needed, adjustment of behavioral goals should be negotiated with clients to fit their preferences and lifestyle needs. Positive reinforcement for making small steps toward behavior change is recommended.

Evaluate the Effectiveness of Teaching Self-Management Skills
Behavior modification helps the client learn and practice new skills, such as eating a healthy diet, exercising and maintaining a healthy weight. Prevention of relapse and providing intervention are important components of a behavior modification program.

It is usually most effective to target a single behavior change at one time and to encourage progress in small steps toward the goal.

Behavioral contracts with clients help establish goals and provide a basis for evaluation. Clients should be assisted in developing goals that they feel are realistic, manageable and measurable.

Examples of measurable goals are:
- I will eat 5 servings of vegetables every day.
- I will walk for 20 minutes 5 days per week.

Clients should set a date for achieving stepwise progress toward a goal. While this should be evaluated at every diabetes visit, intermittent contact can take place over the phone or by email to evaluate clients' self-management skills.

Evaluating the Effectiveness of Education
Educational sessions should be planned to allow adequate time to evaluate client learning. Evaluation of teaching includes asking clients if they have understood the information given and how they could put it into practice. Evaluation can include asking clients if they have further questions or if they found something difficult to understand. Clients can also be asked to summarize the teaching sessions by stating 2 or 3 points that they feel are the most important.

Although tests or quizzes are not inappropriate, they are not always necessary for effective evaluation. Adult learners tend to remember information that is practical and can be readily put to use. Simply asking questions oriented to everyday problem-solving can provide adequate evaluation of learning. An example of a question to evaluate the ability to apply learning could start with "What would you do if..."

Evaluating Client's Psychosocial Adaptation to Diabetes As Result of Education

Healthy coping is identified by the American Association of Diabetes Educators as an outcome of successful diabetes education. Behavioral goals related to this outcome include adaptation to the lifestyle changes required by diabetes and mobilization of an appropriate support system.

Psychosocial adaptation to diabetes involves mastering such behavioral skills as setting realistic goals, solving problems effectively and attaining self-efficacy.

Methods for measuring healthy coping consist of:
- Depression scores, such as the Zung/Beck Depression Scale
- Quality of life measures, such as the Diabetes Quality of Life Measure
- Self-efficacy scales, such as the Diabetes Empowerment Scale
- Self-report of constructs such as self-efficacy, feeling of empowerment, and stress management

An informal or less structured way to assess psychosocial adaptation to diabetes is to ask clients how they feel they are coping. Additionally, clients can be given various scenarios and asked how they would handle them.

Appropriate Documentation of Educational Process

Documentation is a legal requirement of healthcare intervention. It also provides communication between team members and is critical for evaluating outcomes of the diabetes self-management education program.

Documentation is ongoing and must occur at every step of the educational process, which includes assessment, planning, implementation and evaluation of outcomes. Effective documentation is relevant to the individual and his or her goals. Accuracy in documentation ensures legal compliance and effective communication. Documentation should be timely so that results of intervention can be appropriately utilized by other members of the diabetes care team.

Standardized checklists are often used for documenting many of the steps of the educational process. Documentation of each step includes:
- Assessment – identifying the individual's specific learning needs
- Planning – identifying desired outcomes and goals and developing a collaborative plan with the client
- Implementation – describing the educational and behavioral interventions that are designed to help the client achieve the stated goals
- Evaluation – reporting the outcomes of the interventions in relation to the goals

Relevant Services and Healthcare Providers

Community services
- Food stamps, Meals on Wheels, community nutrition sites and centers on aging: Alleviation of risk factors for poor nutrition in elderly clients
- State, local or private rehabilitative services for the blind: Assistance for clients with vision impairment
- Local smoking cessation programs: Assistance for clients with diabetes who smoke and want to quit

Endocrinologist or diabetologist
- Education for preoperative patients with type 1 diabetes about fluid and insulin management during surgery

Gastroenterologist
- Diabetes-related gastroparesis

Gynecologist
- Diabetes-related female sexual dysfunction

Nephrologist
- A glomerular filtration rate (GFR) of 30 ml/min or less

Orthopedist
- Charcot foot: Unilaterally warm and misshapen; "rocker bottom" foot

Podiatrist
- Foot problems or ulcer in conjunction with peripheral neuropathy and/or peripheral vascular disease

Primary Healthcare Provider
- Exercise prescription (if client is planning more than brisk walking or has complications that may be exacerbated by exercise)
- Preconception counseling
- Preventive services

Registered dietitian
- Medical nutrition therapy (MNT); all clients with diabetes should be referred for MNT.
- Celiac disease (intolerance to gluten)
- Gastroparesis

Urologist
- Male sexual dysfunction

Facilitate Communication for Diabetes Team

The person with diabetes is central to the multidisciplinary diabetes team. In addition to the client and healthcare professionals, the team also includes the client's family, spouse and other significant people. Good communication among team members enhances team cohesion and consensus.

An understanding of the roles of each team member is important. However, role definitions that are rigid and territorial are counterproductive. Members of an interdisciplinary team should allow for shared responsibility and flexibility within a framework of shared expectations. Clients must receive consistent messages and treatment approaches across multidisciplinary lines, requiring team members to share a common philosophy.

Encounters with clients should be carefully documented and otherwise communicated to appropriate team members. Behavioral goals, developed with the client, must be included in communication. Client records often include behavioral contracts that facilitate communication of goals.

Team meetings are an effective method of communication and provide a multidisciplinary approach to problem-solving. If team meetings are not feasible, other methods of communication are necessary, such as phone calls and emails.

Good Team Communication

Diabetes education crosses numerous healthcare disciplines. Team members include nurses, physicians, dietitians, mental health professionals, social workers and psychologists, among others.

The team approach implies that education does not stand alone and that everyone teaches across the continuum. Roles should be defined collaboratively and communicated openly because there is considerable overlap of responsibility. Team members' roles may be defined by credentials, areas of expertise or job description.

Examples of role responsibility include:
- Client: Always the center of the team.
- Physician: Establishes diagnosis and guides implementation of medical treatment plan.
- Nurse educator: Coordinates team effort. Also provides self-management education and acute problem management
- Dietitian: Provides nutrition assessment and MNT.
- Mental health and social services professionals: Identify psychosocial barriers and sources of support within the community and family.

Information from the various team members must be consistent, requiring them to communicate what they have told clients. This is true for both oral and written information. When team members provide consistent messages, the client is able to develop trust.

Social Support for the Adolescent

Diabetes educators should be familiar with services tailored to teens that are offered by the American Diabetes Association (ADA), the Juvenile Diabetes Research Foundation (JDRF) and diabetes camps throughout the United States.

Content of diabetes self-management education for the teenager should be relevant to the developmental issues of this stage in life. These issues include peer allegiance, sexuality and contraception, substance abuse, driving issues and social situations. Because peer influences are important, classes and support groups exclusively for teens are appropriate. These groups are most effective when the learning is centered on an activity that is fun.

Diabetes camps facilitate formal and informal learning among the peer group. Learning and sharing with other teens having the same problems and challenges helps develop feelings of normalcy and facilitates problem-solving.

Peer-centered weight loss groups and camps can also benefit the overweight teen with type 2 diabetes.

Assessment Data When Developing Education Program

In order for a diabetes education program to be relevant, it is important to assess the specific needs of the target population. An effective assessment identifies the high priority problems pertinent to the population and addresses their unique characteristics, lifestyle issues and challenges. Thorough assessment reveals the group's barriers to education and self-care, allowing for appropriate program modifications.

Assessment information can be gathered from clients, medical records, focus groups, community forums or the referring healthcare providers.

Examples of items to include in a target-population assessment include:
- Psychosocial attributes
- Cultural characteristics and primary language
- Age and developmental stage
- Physical limitations (e.g., older age or immobility)
- The practice setting (e.g., inpatient, community clinic, HMO)
- Functional limitations
- Educational level
- Economic characteristics
- Barriers to access (e.g., working hours, transportation issues)

Components of Curriculum Development

Curriculum development begins with assessing the needs of the target population. The information gained can be synthesized to create a program relevant to the needs of the participants.

Curriculum development involves prioritizing those needs to fit the timeframe allowed. Safety and survival skills should always be taught first when time is limited.

Curriculum development includes attention to the cultural characteristics of the learners. Language needs should be addressed. Written materials should not only be translated, but modified to be culturally appropriate.

Principles of adult learning should be incorporated into programs for this population. Adults prefer information that is practical and immediately useful. Therefore, the curriculum should emphasize application of knowledge over theoretical information.

Targeting outcomes is an essential element of program development. According the American Association of Diabetes Educators (AADE), behavior change is the focused outcome measurement of diabetes self-management education. Therefore, learning objectives should be stated in measurable behavioral terms.

Goal Setting in an Educational Program

The goals of a diabetes self-management education program must be individualized to the client and relevant to the practice setting where education will take place.

For a patient who is hospitalized with a new diagnosis of diabetes, the goals of education will concentrate on immediate "survival skills" and discharge planning.

These skills include:
- Self-monitoring of blood glucose
- Use of insulin, as appropriate, and insulin actions
- Prevention, detection and treatment of hypoglycemia
- Meal planning

For a patient who has had repeated hospitalizations for diabetic ketoacidosis (DKA) or a history of poor glycemic control, the goals of education are based on the results of a targeted assessment which identifies the areas of need for the individual.

Appropriate program goals for clients who are stable and seen on a continuing outpatient basis are comprehensive. In addition to mastery of survival skills, comprehensive program goals are related to physical activity, weight management, prevention of complications, problem-solving, coping skills, cardiovascular health and other topics for long-term management.

Diabetes Self-Management Education Content Areas

An approved diabetes education program includes basic content areas that have been jointly identified by the ADA and AADE. Content areas were selected based upon evidence that knowledge of these topics has helped people with diabetes achieve favorable outcomes.

Educators should select educational content that matches the needs of the individual or group receiving the education. A learning needs assessment determines how a program should be tailored to such characteristics as age, culture, educational level, type of diabetes and identified learning needs.

Identified content areas for diabetes education include:
- Diabetes disease process and treatment
- Nutritional management
- Physical activity and exercise
- Benefit and use of medication
- Monitoring blood sugar
- Prevention and treatment of acute complications
- Prevention and treatment of chronic complications
- Management of psychosocial issues
- Promotion of health behavior change

ADA Educators 7 Self-Care Behaviors

The American Association of Diabetes Educators (AADE) has identified 7 client-centered areas of self-care behavior needed for successful management of diabetes. This framework for diabetes self-management education is called the AADE7. The self-care behaviors identified by the AADE7 are:

- Healthy eating
- Being physically active
- Monitoring blood glucose and other clinical markers of health
- Taking medication
- Problem-solving
- Healthy coping
- Reducing risk

The impetus for developing the AADE7 was to provide an evidence-based structure for facilitating behavior change and measuring the clinical and health-related outcomes of education. Adopting the AADE7 makes educators accountable for providing interventions that result in measurable improvements in health status, quality of life and healthcare costs. The AADE recommends that educators measure the AADE7 self-care behaviors at both pre-intervention and post-intervention.

Adopting the AADE7 provides grounds for better communication among members of the diabetes education team, allows for comparative research between different self-management education programs and clarifies the processes and outcomes of diabetes self-management education.

Implementation of Diabetes Education Program

Most diabetes education programs take place in group settings, requiring accessible and adequate classroom space. At least one family member or significant other should be allowed to attend classes with the client, so space is needed to accommodate guests. Rooms can be set up in classroom, horseshoe arrangement or another style according to the space available and the needs of the class.

Financial resources will dictate the choices available for audiovisual teaching aids. PowerPoint presentations using a computer and LCD projector can be effective audiovisual tools. Other options include overhead projectors, videotapes, flipcharts and whiteboard with markers.

Other teaching supplies may include participant books, supplemental handouts, pens, notepaper, food models, posters and other teaching models.

A diabetes education program also requires office resources for program planning, storage, communications and documentation. Some programs require an area for seeing clients individually.

Educational Program Adaption to Physical Disabilities

The educator should not assume that clients with physical disabilities are less capable of diabetes self-management or that they are learning disabled. Many people with disabilities are able to effectively manage their diabetes when given the appropriate adaptations in education and equipment. Community and professional organizations can help with planning educational programs adapted to specific disabilities. Examples include the Amputation Coalition of America, the National Association for the Deaf and the American Council for the Blind.

The Americans with Disabilities Act was established to ensure that people with disabilities have the same opportunities and access to services as those without disabilities. For an educator, this means that diabetes self-management education must be accessible to people with disabilities. This may include wheelchair access to classrooms or providing American Sign Language interpreters for educational sessions. Provisions for including those who assist the disabled person should also be incorporated into the teaching plan.

Teaching Methods for the Older Adult

Normal changes in aging can affect the ability to assimilate new information. In addition, comorbidities, such as sensory loss and chronic medical conditions, are common in the elderly client. Teaching sessions should be adapted to these variables.

The pace of teaching should be reduced to accommodate slower processing time. Needs assessment is important in identifying priorities. Teaching sessions should focus on 1 or 2 main points and remain brief.

Reading material should be in print that is easy to read. Blue and green print is often difficult for older people to distinguish. A magnifier should be available for those who need it.

Audio material and verbal instructions should be clear and concise. Use gestures and visual aids to reinforce verbal instructions. Do not assume a hearing impaired person is mentally confused.

Memory aids can help with medication and blood glucose testing adherence. Pill boxes, alarms, calendars and reminder systems can all be employed.

Significant others and caregivers should be involved in education whenever possible.

Market Diabetes Education Program

The first step in marketing a program is to identify the primary customers. Although there may be several types of customers, the marketing plan should focus on the customer who has the greatest potential to provide referrals. Key customers may include healthcare providers, insurers, private-paying clients, organizations and others.

The needs of the primary customer must be identified and marketing messages should match those needs.

Many vehicles for promoting programs are available. Newsletters for physicians, hospitals and communities may be in print form or online. General mailings can be sent to physicians and other key customers. Brochures can be placed in physicians' offices, hospital staff lounges, waiting rooms and local markets and pharmacies. Permission should be obtained prior to leaving brochures in these settings. Personal presentations at hospital staff meetings, physician meetings and professional meetings can be used to promote a program. A website is valuable for marketing and has become increasingly important for business marketing.

Demographic Data for Accreditation of Education Program

The American Diabetes Association's Education Recognition Program (ERP) and the American Association of Diabetes Educators' Diabetes Education Accreditation Program (DEAP) are the two accrediting bodies approved by the Centers for Medicare & Medicaid Services (CMS) for the accreditation of diabetes self-management education programs. Both programs are based on principles of the National Standards for Diabetes Self-Management Education. The accreditation process is similar for both organizations, but each organization has slightly different requirements.

Among other criteria, both the ADA and AADE's programs require tracking and documentation of program and site demographics. The total number of clients who receive education during the data period must be documented, along with the average number of hours of instruction received per client. Follow-up and limited consultation hours must also be documented.

Accredited programs must track and document population statistics such as age, types of diabetes, race and special needs. Program setting and service area characteristics are also included in demographic data. This includes documenting the type of service provided and information about the academic instructors' experience, academic credentials and education.

Health Insurance Portability and Accountability Act

HIPAA is a federal law that protects the privacy of consumers' health information. It applies to oral, written and electronic information and must be followed by health plans and healthcare providers. In the healthcare setting, health information can only be used to the extent that it is needed to provide and coordinate care.

HIPAA requires that healthcare providers have safeguards in place to maintain the security and confidentiality of health information. Employers must provide training programs for employees to demonstrate how information is to be protected.

Insurance companies may legally receive health information in order to settle claims. Public health departments and law enforcement agencies are also allowed access to medical records when appropriate to their duties in protecting and serving society.

Family members and other significant people who are involved in a client's care are allowed access to information only when the client has given permission.

ADA Standards of Care for Adults

Self monitoring of blood glucose:
Valuable for virtually all clients with diabetes. Those requiring intensive insulin therapy should monitor at least 3 times per day.

The A1C test:
Should be performed at least 2 times per year in clients with glycemic control. It should be performed quarterly in those not meeting glycemic goals and as needed for making decisions about changes in treatment.

Glycemic goal:
An A1C < 7% is the goal for most adults.

Medical nutrition therapy (MNT):
Clients with prediabetes and diabetes should receive comprehensive MNT provided by a registered dietitian. Diet should meet recommended dietary allowances for all micronutrients.

Weight loss for overweight and obese people:
Modest weight loss by following a low-carbohydrate or low-fat, calorie-restricted diet, along with exercise and behavior modification, is recommended.

Primary prevention of diabetes:
For the prevention of diabetes in those with high risk, modest weight loss, increased physical activity and a diet with plenty of fiber and whole grain foods is recommended.

Saturated fat intake:
Should be less than 7% of total caloric intake.

Carbohydrate intake:
Should be monitored by carbohydrate counting, exchanges or experience-based estimation.

Non-nutritive sweeteners and sugar alcohols:
Are safe when consumed within limitations set by the Food and Drug Administration.

Routine supplementation with antioxidants and chromium:
There is insufficient evidence to recommend routine supplementation with vitamin A, vitamin C, carotene or chromium.

Bariatric surgery:
Should be considered for individuals with diabetes who have a BMI > 35, along with lifestyle support and medical monitoring.

Diabetes self-management education:
A program meeting national standards should be available to all people with diabetes upon diagnosis and as needed thereafter. Education should address psychosocial and emotional needs.

Physical activity:
At least 150 minutes per week of moderate intensity aerobic exercise and resistance training 3 times per week.

Psychosocial assessment and care:
Should be included as an ongoing part of diabetes care.

Hypoglycemia:
Treatment with 15 – 20 grams of glucose is preferred, although other forms of glucose-containing carbohydrate may be used. Glucagon should be prescribed for those at risk for severe hypoglycemia. Those with hypoglycemic unawareness should modify glycemic targets to avoid hypoglycemia.

Immunization:
Annual influenza vaccine is recommended for all people with diabetes who are over the age of 6 months. Pneumococcal vaccine is recommended for all people with diabetes who are over age 2. Revaccination is recommended for those over age 64 if the initial vaccine was administered over 5 years ago.

Hypertension:
Measure blood pressure (BP) at every routine visit. Goal is less than 130/80 mmHg. Clients with BP greater than 140/80 should receive pharmacologic therapy, usually beginning with an ACE inhibitor or angiotensin receptor blocker (ARB).

Dyslipidemia:
Measure fasting lipid profile at least annually. Goals are:
- LDL less than 100 mg/dl
- HDL greater than 50 mg/dl
- Triglycerides less than 150 mg/dl

Antiplatelet agents:
For primary prevention of cardiovascular disease (CVD), 75 – 162 mg of aspirin per day should be considered for most men over 50 years of age and most women over 60 who have at least one additional risk factor. Aspirin is used as secondary prevention in people with a history of CVD. Clopidogrel may be substituted.

Smoking cessation:
Advise clients not to smoke and provide cessation counseling as part of routine care.

Coronary heart disease:
Evaluate risk in asymptomatic clients by 10-year risk and treat accordingly. In clients with known CVD, therapy with ACE inhibitor, aspirin and statin is indicated. Beta blockers should be used for at least 2 years following a cardiovascular event.

Nephropathy:
Optimize blood glucose and blood pressure control to reduce the risk or slow the progression of nephropathy. Screen urine albumin and serum creatinine at least annually. Treatment with ACE inhibitors or ARBs is recommended for non-pregnant clients with albuminuria.

Retinopathy:
Optimize blood glucose and blood pressure control to reduce the risk or slow the progression of retinopathy. Perform initial dilated eye exam soon after diagnosis of type 2 diabetes and 5 years after onset of type 1. Repeat annually or more often if retinopathy is progressing. Those with glycemic control may repeat dilated eye exam every 2 – 3 years following 1 or more normal exams.

Neuropathy:
Screen for distal symmetrical neuropathy upon diagnosis of diabetes and at least annually thereafter. Screen for cardiovascular autonomic neuropathy upon diagnosis of type 2 diabetes and after 5 years of onset of type 1.

Foot care:
Annual comprehensive foot exam should include inspection, palpation of pulses and testing for loss of protective sensation. Sensory testing should include monofilament test and vibratory sense, pinprick sensation or ankle reflexes. Provide foot care education to all clients with diabetes.

ADA Standards of Care for Children and Adolescents

Hypertension:
- Blood pressure (BP) consistently above the 90th percentile for age, sex and height should first be treated with lifestyle modification.
- Pharmacological intervention is indicated if goals are not achieved in 3 – 6 months. ACE inhibitors are considered first-line therapy.
- BP goal is less than 130/80 or below the 90th percentile, whichever is lower.

Dyslipidemia:
- Fasting lipid profile is indicated for any child greater than 2 years of age with family history of hypercholesterolemia or early cardiovascular event. In the absence of risk factors, screening for dyslipidemia should be performed on any child with diabetes who is 10 years or older.
- Target is LDL less than 100 mg/dl.
- Initial treatment is with lifestyle modification emphasizing the reduction of saturated fat in the diet.

Treatment with a statin medication is indicated in children greater than 10 years old having LDL greater than 160 mg/dl. In the presence of cardiovascular risk factors, statins are recommended when the LDL is greater than 130 mg/dl.

Infection Control Practices

Handwashing facilities should be available in areas where insulin injection or fingerstick techniques are being practiced. Occupational Safety and Health Administration (OSHA) and Joint Commission on Accreditation of Healthcare Organizations (JCAHCO) requirements should be consulted for procedures to appropriately clean of areas where blood products are used.

Clients do not usually need to use alcohol swabs to disinfect the skin prior to pricking the finger or injecting insulin. Handwashing and good personal hygiene are normally adequate. Alcohol may be used to cleanse the skin when handwashing facilities are not available or when the insulin injection site is unclean.

Educators should be knowledgeable about local requirements for syringe and lancet disposal. Many areas have regulations requiring that medical sharps be disposed of as hazardous waste. Disposing of containers with used sharps in bins designated for recycling is prohibited.

While manufactures do not recommend the reuse of needles and lancets, the American Diabetes Association (ADA) does not forbid it. Clients with acute concurrent illness, compromised immunity or poor personal hygiene should not reuse needles.

Measurable Health Outcomes

Health outcomes are measurable changes in a person's condition resulting from healthcare intervention over time. Medicare and Medicaid Services, policymakers and professional accrediting bodies all rely on outcomes data to assess the quality of interventions and the delivery of healthcare.

Baseline data must be available for interventions in order for them to be evaluated. Without a baseline, change cannot be demonstrated.

There are different types of measurable outcomes. These include:
- Clinical outcomes – changes in biological measures such as A1C, blood pressure and lipids
- Education outcomes – changes in knowledge or skills
- Quality of life (QOL) outcomes – changes in measures of QOL, such as the SF-36 and PAID questionnaire
- Behavioral outcomes – changes in such behaviors as physical activity or food choices
- Cost-effectiveness – the cost of the program versus its cost savings from improved health

Appropriate Program Outcomes for Diabetes Self-Management Education

Outcomes demonstrate changes in health status as a result of an intervention. There are different kinds of outcomes, such as clinical, education and psychosocial.

The American Association of Diabetes Educators (AADE) Outcomes Task Force has concluded that health-related behaviors are the unique and measurable outcomes for diabetes education. The AADE7 identifies the diabetes self-care behaviors as:
- Being physically active
- Healthy eating
- Taking medication
- Self-monitoring
- Problem-solving
- Reducing risk for complications
- Healthy coping

Measurable changes in these behaviors from the baseline demonstrate the effectiveness of a diabetes education program. Recognition of these behavioral outcomes has changed the focus of the diabetes education curriculum from being content-driven to outcomes-driven.

Valid outcomes require a baseline, or pre-program, measurement. This is followed by measurement at regular intervals and post-program. Aggregate population outcomes are pooled outcomes from many different individuals. Aggregate outcomes guide the program and are used in the continuous quality-improvement process.

Continuous Quality Improvement

CQI is one of the most widely used methodologies for supporting service excellence and customer satisfaction. It has been adopted by the American Diabetes Association (ADA) Recognition Program as a requirement for accreditation of diabetes self-management education programs.

CQI is an overriding business philosophy that applies to daily operations. Successful CQI programs have the buy-in of all staff, not just the managers. CQI is a proactive process that employs systems for preventive management on a daily basis as opposed to relying on crisis management when things are not done right the first time.

Problem identification is an important part of the CQI process. Problems are often considered opportunities for improvement. Data about the problem is systematically collected and analyzed to generate possible solutions. After implementation of a recommended solution, quality outcomes are evaluated and improvement is measured.

Public Screening for Diabetes

The appropriateness of performing random fingerstick blood glucose testing to screen for diabetes at community health fairs, shopping malls and other public places is questionable. Blood glucose results collected in this way are difficult to evaluate and may not be accurate or reliable. Further, this practice has not been demonstrated to be cost-effective. For these reasons, the American Diabetes Association (ADA) does not recommend community blood glucose testing to screen for diabetes.

However, public screening for diabetes risk by other means is advocated. This involves risk-factor assessment by a health professional to identify those at high risk for type 2 diabetes and cardiovascular disease. High-risk people can be made aware of their risk and referred to a healthcare provider for blood glucose testing. As a public health benefit, this may result in early detection and treatment and promotes preventive strategies.

Legal Rights in the Workplace

Diabetes educators must be knowledgeable about clients' legal rights in the workplace and be prepared to advocate for them. The law protects people with diabetes from job discrimination based solely upon having diabetes and includes being allowed reasonable accommodations to enable diabetes management.

The Americans with Disabilities Act Amendments Act (ADAAA) of 2008 protects people with diabetes from discrimination in the workplace. The law requires that people with diabetes be afforded reasonable accommodations to follow a doctor's orders and protects them from being fired as long as they can perform the essential functions of the job. For example, a person on insulin may require a break at a particular time to be able to eat and avoid hypoglycemia.

A letter from a healthcare provide to the employer can explain the client's need for reasonable workplace accommodations and fulfill the requirements of the ADAAA to protect the client's job security. The letter should document how diabetes affects major life activities and describe the reasonable accommodations needed for the client's self-management.

Practice Test

Practice Questions

1. What is the first step in the process of diabetes self-management education?
    A. Assessment
    B. Goal setting
    C. Diagnosis
    D. Referral

2. Which of the following options is an outcome of personal record keeping in relation to physical activity, according to recent studies?
    A. Those who keep logs of physical activity are more adherent to other elements of therapy (i.e. diet, medication)
    B. Those who keep exercise logs are more likely to enroll in organized exercise programs (i.e. gym memberships, classes, etc.)
    C. Keeping a physical activity log is associated with a higher level of self efficacy
    D. The obligation of record keeping has been identified as a barrier to exercise by study participants

3. Consider the following patient: male, age 46, previously sedentary, mild hypertension and hyperlipidemia (both adequately controlled with medication), type 2 diabetes, and a BMI of 26. If this patient wishes to begin a moderate-intensity exercise regimen, what additional assessment may be warranted?
    A. Stress test with ECG (electrocardiogram)
    B. DEXA scan to assess bone density and strength
    C. Ankle-brachial index to rule out peripheral arterial disease
    D. None, as BP and cholesterol are being controlled and exercise is only moderate intensity

4. In your role as diabetes educator for a clinic, you both assess and instruct patients on a variety of self-care skills. Which teaching strategy provides the best opportunity to both assess *and* instruct on *self-administration of insulin*?
    A. A written quiz in which the patient puts insulin administration steps in order
    B. A demonstration and return demonstration of insulin administration
    C. A video that can be viewed and reviewed on proper insulin administration technique
    D. A printed handout with pictures depicting steps of insulin administration, followed by verbal acknowledgement of understanding

5. The following policies are part of your DSME program: asking patients if there are any dietary preferences or restrictions; inviting family members to participate; and being sensitive to your rate of speech and tone of voice. These policies address which specific type of consideration?
    A. Readiness for change variation among your patients
    B. Potential low literacy/numeracy levels among your patients
    C. Cultural characteristics/barriers of your population
    D. Poor family and social support

6. According to the ADA consensus statement on managing preexisting diabetes for pregnancy (2008), what is the optimal glycemic target for pregnant women with preexisting diabetes (assuming the target may be reached without excessive hypoglycemia)?
    A. Pre-meal/fasting glucose: 60 to 90 mg/dL; peak postprandial: <120 mg/dL; A1c <5.5%
    B. Pre-meal/fasting glucose: 60 to 99 mg/dL; peak postprandial: <129 mg/dL; A1c <6%
    C. Pre-meal/fasting glucose: 70 to 100 mg/dL; peak postprandial: <120 mg/dL; A1c <6.5%
    D. Pre-meal/fasting glucose: 70 to 110 mg/dL; peak postprandial: <140 mg/dL; A1c <7%

7. During the initial assessment process, your patient answers the question, "How important is it for you to make this change right now?" with a 9 out of 10 (very important) and answers the question, "How confident are you that you will be able to make this change?" with a 2 out of 10 (not very important). In customizing her DSME plan, what should your focus be?
    A. Providing materials and experiences to enhance her knowledge and skills
    B. Addressing psychosocial needs, such as accepting her diagnosis and managing stress levels
    C. Highlighting the benefits of good diabetes management as a way to encourage behavior change
    D. Explaining the two questions further to confirm understanding, as it is very uncommon for a patient to rate the readiness-to-change elements this far apart.

8. It is important to assess potential barriers to self-monitoring of blood glucose, especially for patients who are not adhering to their plan of care recommendations. Which of the following barriers was *not* one cited by patients in recent studies?
    A. Cost of testing supplies
    B. Discomfort of finger sticks
    C. Lack of instruction and support
    D. Misplacement of small items

9. When assessing for risk of hypoglycemia in relation to exercise, which element of the patient record is most important to consider?
    A. The patient's typical signs and symptoms with hypoglycemia
    B. Current patient physical/glycemic status (wt., BMI, A1c)
    C. Timing and content (i.e. carb content) of meals in relation to the activity
    D. Medication regimen: types, dose, and timing

10. Which of the following behaviors is the *most* likely indication that the patient is at a very low level of readiness to change?
    A. The patient becomes tearful as you explain how to keep a food diary
    B. The patient watches your demonstration but does not say anything
    C. The patient volunteers to answer a review question at the end of class but gets the answer totally wrong
    D. The patient denies that she has diabetes and disagrees with the doctor's referral for DSME

11. According to ADA Standards, which statement is *not* true regarding medical nutrition therapy and diabetes?
   A. Medical nutrition therapy is recommended for only those persons with diabetes who are underweight, overweight, or obese.
   B. Medical nutrition therapy is recommended for anyone who has diabetes, regardless of nutritional status.
   C. Children with diabetes and celiac disease should consult with a registered dietitian familiar with both conditions.
   D. Because nutrition in the hospital setting is complex, a registered dietitian should be part of the inpatient diabetes care team to provide medical nutrition therapy.

12. You are assessing a patient's blood glucose monitoring technique by having her demonstrate a blood glucose test. Which of the following actions is indicative of *improper* technique?
   A. Cleaning her hands with warm water and soap instead of alcohol
   B. Setting the lancet device to her preference
   C. Milking the lanced finger at the tip to acquire a sufficient blood sample
   D. Recording the reading in her notebook rather than on the clinic-provided sheet

13. Your patient suffers from obesity, type 2 diabetes, hypertension, and hyperlipidemia. He recalls his dinner from last night: a low-fat turkey and cheese sandwich with mustard, a side salad with low-fat Italian dressing, pickles, a small serving of baked chips, and one can of club soda. Based on your assessment, which of the patient's conditions is at *greatest* risk due to his food choices?
   A. Hyperlipidemia
   B. Type 2 diabetes
   C. Obesity
   D. Hypertension

14. A patient with gestational diabetes (GDM) is convinced she developed GDM from eating too much of her favorite food – popcorn – early in her pregnancy. She insists that if she does not eat any again during her pregnancy, she will not have to start insulin and her blood glucose values will return to normal. What emotional stage associated with chronic disease diagnosis (similar to Kubler-Ross stages of grief) do you assess in your patient?
   A. Denial
   B. Anger
   C. Bargaining
   D. Frustration & depression

15. Which instructional strategy is likely to be *most* effective in terms of patient retention?
   A. PowerPoint presentation with funny visuals and bullet list of main points
   B. Current, well-referenced booklets with colorful diagrams, written at a patient's optimal reading level, that can be reviewed as desired
   C. One-on-one conversation over the phone where the educator presents information and then rephrases the information using analogies to ensure understanding
   D. Small group discussion around a table where patients teach each other a skill after seeing it explained and demonstrated by the educator

16. Of the choices below, what is the strongest predictor of health status?
    A. Ethnic group
    B. Literacy skill
    C. Income level
    D. Age

17. Your patient, a 29-year-old Hispanic female, tells you her goal is to lose 15 lbs. by her wedding day in three months. What element of the nutrition assessment is most important to focus on to help her meet her goal?
    A. Composition of nutrients (protein/fat vs. carbohydrates)
    B. Energy balance (total calorie intake vs. expenditure)
    C. Type and amounts of carbohydrates consumed (i.e. glycemic index)
    D. Total grams of fiber per day

18. Which of the following assessment items is *not* considered a component of the "knowledge" area?
    A. Literacy/numeracy
    B. Level of family support
    C. Previous diabetes self-management education
    D. Proficiency of self-care skills

19. Which of the following does *not* need to be noted on the medication regimen portion of the initial DSME assessment?
    A. Daily multiple vitamin with iron
    B. Two cinnamon capsules with each meal
    C. Emergency albuterol inhaler for asthma (but has not used in three years)
    D. All of the above should be noted

20. An adult male patient who is 6'1", 215 lbs., and with type 2 diabetes, completes a 24-hour dietary recall. Which of his meals, reported below, do you assess to be the one *most* in need of modification?
    A. Breakfast: 1 cup of Raisin Bran cereal with 1 cup skim milk, 12 oz. orange juice, $\frac{1}{2}$ bagel
    B. Lunch: Large taco salad (tortilla bowl, chicken, cheese, lettuce, tomato, salsa, refried beans, sour cream), 16 oz. Diet Coke
    C. Dinner: 2 cheese burgers (with lean beef), side salad with light Italian dressing, 1 cup green beans, black coffee
    D. All meals are equally inappropriate and in need of modification

21. When asked about his personal goal for diabetes education, your patient's reply is, "I don't know what you mean." What would be an appropriate response?
    A. "What do you mean you don't know what I mean?"
    B. "How do you hope that learning more about diabetes will help you?"
    C. Do not say anything; allow him to think longer and then respond to you
    D. "Well, for example, would you like to achieve your ideal weight, or reach your target blood sugar? You know, things like that."

22. A patient who has identified himself as a visual learner would likely most prefer which method of instruction?
   A. Role-playing a scenario in which he orders a balanced meal at a restaurant
   B. Seeing pictures of food portions followed by booklets on meal planning
   C. A spoken explanation of how to adjust insulin depending on pre-meal glucose
   D. Group discussion on challenges relating to dealing with the stress of diabetes

23. You are reading the patient chart of a 30-year old African-American female, newly diagnosed with diabetes (type is unspecified). Her body mass index (BMI) is recorded as 17.5 kg.m2. Her BMI falls into which category?
   A. Underweight
   B. Normal weight
   C. Overweight
   D. Obese

24. What is the *main* purpose of personal record keeping with regards to dietary habits?
   A. The patient is able to look back and feel proud for the positive changes that have been made, thus promoting patient empowerment.
   B. A food record allows the patient and educator to review, evaluate, and reassess choices, which can be used to set or modify nutritional goals.
   C. Insurance providers need to see evidence of the impact of medical nutrition therapy (MNT) and the food record can be admitted as part of the official patient record.
   D. Keeping a food record forces the patient to pay more attention to what he or she is eating, and promotes the important diabetes life skill of recording daily activities.

25. Which hypothetical situation would you pose if you wanted to assess a patient's ability to deal with a glucose emergency?
   A. You are shopping for items for a special birthday meal that will also fit into your diabetes meal plan. What would you choose?
   B. What actions would you take if you were traveling out of state and realized on your trip that you were almost out of insulin?
   C. Say you are driving your car and you begin to feel shaky, sweaty, and confused. What would you do?
   D. How would you deal with a colleague who found out you have diabetes and proceeded to give you advice you knew to be incorrect?

26. You assess a patient's self-administration of insulin with a non-refillable insulin pen device and a 5 mm pen needle. The patient performs the following actions: clean the end of the pen with alcohol, attach the pen needle, dial the dose, insert the needle into the skin and fully press the button, withdraw after 10 seconds, detach and dispose of the needle, replace the pen cap. What was incorrect about the way the patient performed this skill?
   A. He needed to clean the skin with alcohol
   B. He needed to pinch the skin before injecting
   C. He left the pen needle in the skin for 10 seconds after injecting insulin
   D. He needed to prime the needle before dialing the dose

27. In a discussion on meal planning, your patient states, "My whole family is from Mexico, and they get offended when I don't want to eat our traditional foods." What type of barrier do you assess this patient is facing?
   A. Physical barrier related to problem solving
   B. Interpersonal barrier related to healthy eating
   C. Personal independence barrier related to healthy coping
   D. Financial barrier related to personal independence and family relationships

28. Which theoretical approach to learning and health behavioral change theory maintains that individuals learn from their personal experiences as well as from observing the actions and experiences of others?
   A. Social Cognitive Theory (SCT)
   B. Health Belief Model (HBM)
   C. Theory of Planned Behavior (TPB)
   D. Transtheoretical Model (TTM)

29. Which of the following has *not* been identified as a major barrier to care, according to the 2006 "Barriers to Optimal Care for Patients with Diabetes and Strategies to Overcome Them?"
   A. Low level of health literacy
   B. Lack of interest on the part of patients
   C. Limited time to see the provider
   D. Complexity of diabetes education

30. Which of the following patient statements represents a situation in which specialty care provider resources are *not* being used according to ADA recommendations?
   A. "I see a dentist twice a year even though I do not have, and have never had, gum disease."
   B. I see my ophthalmologist annually even though he says that I have no signs of retinopathy."
   C. I have my cholesterol checked every year even though my LDL, HDL, and triglyceride levels have always been within normal limits."
   D. "I see a nephrologist annually even though my BP is normal and I have no diagnosed kidney problems."

31. How frequently should a diabetes educator assess a patient's tobacco use status and readiness-to-quit status?
   A. At every visit for those patients who smoke and only at the initial assessment for those who do not.
   B. Annually, unless the patient brings it up (smoking status or readiness to quit)
   C. At every visit
   D. Whenever the educator notes signs that indicate a possible change in status

32. Which of the following assessment findings is most likely to indicate poor circulation in the lower extremities?
   A. Substantial hair on the tops of the toes
   B. Ankle-brachial index of 1.0
   C. Diminished dorsalis pedal pulses
   D. Positive pinprick sensation at the level of the ankle

33. Your patient, an older gentleman with type 2 diabetes, reports exercising six days per week: 40 min. of jogging on M/W/F and 40 minutes of strength training on T/Th/Sa. As part of your assessment, you should consider whether which type of physical activity recommendation is being addressed?
  A. Aerobic exercise
  B. Toning exercise
  C. Flexibility exercise
  D. Resistance exercise

34. Which of the following examples would you assess to be the *most* appropriate example of SMBG record keeping?
  A. A patient records her BG values with time, date, medications, food intake, and other activities in a spiral notebook instead of the log sheet provided by the clinic. The book is tattered and stained with blood and food.
  B. A patient simply allows the meter to record all readings, which he then brings to the clinic for each visit.
  C. A patient does not bring her meter to the clinic but writes her BG values on the log sheet provided by the clinic. She lists only the values and no other information (food, activity, medication).
  D. A patient writes his BG values in the logbook that came with his meter. He includes times, activity levels, and illnesses, but does not write dates, food intake, or medication doses on the pages. He admits that he just picks any blank page to start the week and that some are out of order.

35. As part of the initial comprehensive DSME assessment, you ask your patient to describe his meals and snacks from the past 24 hours. He states that he cannot recall what he ate yesterday. What action or response would be *most* appropriate?
  A. Note, "Pt. does not recall" in your documentation and move on to the next question.
  B. Invite his wife, who has accompanied him, to help recall what he ate yesterday.
  C. Give the participant a 24-hour dietary log sheet and ask him to return it completed by next week.
  D. Encourage him by prompting, "Now, Honey, I can't believe that a man as smart as you can't come up with anything..."

36. You are reviewing recent lab data for a new patient with diabetes but with no other documented co-morbidities. Which lab value is of the greatest concern?
  A. Hemoglobin A1c of 7.8%
  B. LDL of 101 mg/dL
  C. HDL of 88 mg/dL
  D. Serum creatinine of 2.8 mg/dL

37. When asked to explain to you why he takes a specific oral diabetes medication, the patient does not look at the label. Instead, he opens the bottle and takes out a pill. Which possible barrier should you investigate further?
  A. Financial
  B. Cognitive
  C. Health literacy
  D. Fear of side effects

38. What is *acanthosis nigricans* and what does it suggest?
   A. A darkening and thickening of the skin, typically on the back/sides of the neck or the axillae; indicative of insulin resistance
   B. A pattern of deep, labored breathing; indicative of acidosis, common in advanced DKA
   C. Darkening of the toe nails; indicative of poor pedal circulation
   D. Blackening around the edges of an ulcer; indicative of tissue ischemia due to poor circulation and oxygenation

39. Which of the following methods is *least* recommended as a valid way to perform an initial patient DSME assessment?
   A. Talking to the nurse of the referring provider and using the information to complete the assessment form
   B. Meeting with the patient face-to-face and asking questions of the patient and his spouse
   C. Having patients complete an assessment form online before the first appointment and then following up with a few questions in person
   D. Observing patients in a group setting while having each member of the group complete personal information on a standardized assessment form

40. Which patient statement regarding medication administration would cause you to suspect further education is needed?
   A. "When I had to skip breakfast and lunch the day of my procedure, I took my Diabeta® (glyburide) but skipped my Levemir® (detemir)."
   B. "I leave my Lantus pen on my nightstand all the time so I will remember to take it at bedtime."
   C. "I take my metformin every morning, even if I will be skipping breakfast."
   D. "I throw away the NovoLog® (aspart) vial of insulin I am using after four weeks, even if it is still half full."

41. Which of the following patient statements would be *least* important to note in the health history section of the initial DSME assessment?
   A. "My mother believes I got diabetes from eating too much candy as a kid."
   B. "I was hospitalized eight months ago for DKA."
   C. "I experience low blood sugar episodes about twice a month."
   D. "I have had diabetes for 4 years, but I am not sure what type I have."

42. Which of the following choices is *not* information to be gathered as part of the initial individual DSME assessment, according to the ADA National Standards for DSME (2013)?
   A. Financial status
   B. Emotional response to diabetes
   C. Cultural and religious practices that could affect diabetes
   D. Sexual orientation

43. Which of the following patients would be classified as "morbidly obese"?
   A. A 50-year-old white male who is 22 kg (about 49 lbs.) overweight and has already suffered one heart attack
   B. A 26-year-old Hispanic female with a BMI of 41 kg/m²
   C. A 48-year-old African-American male who is consulting a specialist for possible bariatric surgery
   D. A 60-year-old white male who weighs 225 lbs (about 102 kg)

44. Which of the following choices would be the *most* appropriate method for screening for patient numeracy challenges?
   A. Ask the patient about the highest grade he or she completed and how well the patient did in math.
   B. Ask the patient if he or she has any trouble doing math problems.
   C. Give the patient a standardized assessment test to be completed at home and have the patient bring it to the next appointment.
   D. Present applicable hypothetical situations, such as choosing a menu with specified total grams of carbs or calculating a mealtime insulin dose using a correction scale.

45. Which of the following items are considered Standards of Care (2013) for adults with Type 1 or Type 2 diabetes?
   A. Annual eye exam and annual echocardiogram
   B. Annual influenza vaccination and dilated eye exam every six months (more often if needed)
   C. Hepatitis B vaccination for adults less than 60 yrs and annual influenza vaccination for all patients
   D. Annual C-peptide lab and A1c lab test every six months (more often if not to goal)

46. According to Medicare guidelines, which of the following patient characteristics or situations is *not* justification for individual sessions of diabetes education (over group sessions)?
   A. The patient prefers one-on-one education because he does not get along with others
   B. No group classes are available within two months of the referral
   C. The patient has visual and or language limitations
   D. The physician has a document request for individual education, based on the educator's assessment and recommendation.

47. A 59 y/o single female patient with type 2 diabetes admits that she only takes half of her recommended Januvia® (sitagliptin) tablet, but does take her full metformin tablet. She later tells you that she has added more vegetables to her meals, but only canned vegetables. Based on these brief statements, what barrier do you believe is *most* likely a concern for this patient?
   A. Transportation barrier
   B. Cultural barrier
   C. Cognitive ability barrier
   D. Financial barrier

48. A patient who is reluctant to attend DSME class states the reason as, "I already know all this stuff." In light of his learning readiness, what would be the *most* appropriate action?
   A. Tell him that if he changes his mind, he may call you at any time. Document his refusal to participate.
   B. Give him a pop quiz with challenging diabetes knowledge questions to help him see that he does not know everything.
   C. Acknowledge his reluctance and ask if he might be willing to share some of his knowledge and experiences with the other class members.
   D. Change the subject to minimize conflict and then speak with his wife to see if she might have better luck convincing him.

49. Which of the following patient statements should alert you to a *lack* of understanding about the purpose of self-monitoring of blood glucose?
    A. "I test my blood sugar whenever I feel bad, even if it is not my regularly scheduled time to test."
    B. "I test two to three times per day and schedule my testing times for when I think my numbers will be the best."
    C. "I wake up at 3:00 in the morning and test for a couple of days whenever my doctor changes my dose of basal insulin."
    D. "I try to test a couple of hours after a meal to see if my mealtime insulin dose was too little or too much."

50. Which of the following is *not* considered a critical skill needed by the diabetes educator to assess patients' abilities to *plan* goals?
    A. Interpret Information Gathering (i.e. assesses attitude, knowledge, and skill related to goal setting ability)
    B. Facilitating Engagement (i.e. uses skills to build a trusting relationship)
    C. Reporting Progress (i.e. documenting past and present progress, or lack thereof, in achieving set goals)
    D. Problem Analysis (i.e. develops an understanding of factors related to a patient's self-management problems)

51. A patient comes into your clinic to sign up for diabetes education classes. He tells you that he has had diabetes for 12 years but did not want to face his diagnosis. Now, after seeing how he is unable to keep up with his grandchildren, he has realized the need to make some changes and control his blood sugar. What stage of change in the transtheoretical model most accurately describes this patient's state?
    A. Precontemplation
    B. Contemplation
    C. Preparation
    D. Action

52. Which of the following is *not* among the top treatment fears for patients who are being prescribed insulin?
    A. Nausea and subsequent weight loss
    B. Worsening of their diabetes
    C. Needles
    D. Hypoglycemia

53. An older patient is not completing her assessment paperwork along with other group members. She moves slowly and squints at the signs on the door. Her hands shake as she retrieves an item from her handbag. Based on what you have briefly observed, which of the following learning barriers do you *most* likely suspect may be present?
    A. Visual and tactile/dexterity
    B. Hearing and literacy
    C. Financial and visual
    D. Mobility and cultural

54. A patient in your DSME group asks why a person cannot use oral medication to treat type 1 diabetes. Which is the most accurate and appropriate response?

    A. "Because type 2 diabetes is brought on by weight, and weight gain is a side effect of insulin, we avoid using insulin in those with type 2 diabetes while we prefer it for those with type 1, who are typically underweight."

    B. "Everyone needs insulin to live. In type 2 diabetes, the insulin–producing cells (beta cells) may still be working somewhat but not well enough to keep blood sugar normal. Oral medications help the body's insulin to work better. In type 1 diabetes, the body has destroyed its own beta cells and so we must use insulin from an outside source."

    C. "Type 1 diabetes is a more severe form of diabetes, and therefore, we go straight for the most potent medication. Type 2 diabetes, on the other hand, is less severe and can be minimized by lifestyle changes, and so there are "less drastic" medication options."

    D. "Because type 2 diabetes is characterized by insulin resistance, most oral medications for type 2 diabetes work by improving a body's sensitivity to insulin. Those with type 1 diabetes are very sensitive to insulin. If some of these oral medications were used to treat someone who has type 1 diabetes, they would likely cause severe hypoglycemia."

55. In relation to safe driving, which of the following advice would the clinician *least* likely recommend?

    A. Always wear medical identification when driving.

    B. When driving long distances, stop every one to two hours to check blood glucose.

    C. Always eat something with carbohydrates within the hour before you drive.

    D. Keep some form of glucose or quick carb handy in the vehicle at all times.

56. Which *active*-learning instructional strategy listed below is one in which the educator has the *most* control over content?

    A. Group discussion

    B. Conversation maps

    C. Lecture with visual aids (i.e. slides)

    D. Demonstration

57. For how long following intense, extended exercise should a person be concerned with the possibility of activity-related hypoglycemia (assuming the person uses insulin)?

    A. Up to 24 hours after the activity

    B. Up to 8 hours after the activity

    C. Up to 4 hours after the activity

    D. Up to 2 hours after the activity

58. The provider for your patient added pioglitazone (Actos®) to the patient's regimen one month ago. Your patient visits you today and says that he is dissatisfied with the new medicine, as it "has not done one thing to help my blood sugar." After acknowledging his frustration, how would you respond to his complaint?

    A. Suggest that he discontinue the medication and ask the provider to try something else

    B. Suggest that a higher dose may be needed and offer to consult with the provider to authorize a higher dose

    C. Suggest that the medicine may not be working because he is likely eating more, as evidenced by his weight gain since the last visit

    D. Explain that medications in this class can take up to 12 weeks to work.

59. Look at the patient statement below. Then select the choice that is the *best* example of "developing discrepancy", one of the guiding principles of motivational interviewing.

Patient: "I just can't stand testing my blood sugar, although I have to admit that when I do and the number is high, I act on it right away."

    A. Educator: "Just be glad that we have the meters we do today. Back in the day, it took more than a minute to get the result and you needed a much bigger drop of blood, which meant a much more painful finger poke!"

    B. Educator: "It sounds like you are dealing with some serious obstacles when it comes to self-monitoring; yet, I also sense that when you do test, you are able to use the information to help you correct high blood sugars when needed. What effect do you think those corrections will have on your health in the long run?"

    C. Educator: "It is just one of those things that people with diabetes have to deal with. Trust me, you are not alone – almost none of my patients enjoy testing their blood sugar, and I tell them the same thing I am telling you."

    D. Educator: "Great job coming in with your meter and log book today. Let's see how you did over the last two weeks on correcting for highs and treating lows."

60. Which of the following mental health conditions that are commonly associated with diabetes can be addressed primarily by the diabetes educator and may *not* necessarily require a referral to a mental health professional?
    A. Depression
    B. Behavioral relapse
    C. Eating disorder (i.e. bulimia)
    D. Anxiety

61. Which of the following exercise precautions applies specifically to patients with *unstable proliferative retinopathy*?
    A. Exercise beyond only what is needed for activities of daily living (slow walking) is not advised, as increased blood flow may exacerbate retinal problems.
    B. Swimming and other prone physical activities should be avoided as they increase pressure in the retinas.
    C. Resistance training should not be included in the exercise regimen because the resulting excessive systolic blood pressure response may further damage the eyes.
    D. Before beginning a moderate-intensity exercise program consisting of both aerobic and strength training exercises, patients should have a stress test and be cleared by a cardiologist.

62. Which of the following medications may react with glipizide (Glucotrol®) in a way that may result in an increased risk for *hypoglycemia*?
    A. Corticosteroids (i.e. Deltasone®*)*
    B. Protease inhibitors (i.e. indinavir)
    C. Estrogen products (i.e. Premarin®)
    D. Sulfonamides (i.e. Bactrim®)

63. Which diabetes medication classes are generally contraindicated for patients with congestive heart failure (CHF)?
   A. DPP-4 inhibitors (i.e. sitagliptin) and alphaglucosidase inhibitors (starch blockers)
   B. Biguanides (i.e. metformin) and TZDs (i.e. pioglitazone)
   C. Sulfonylureas (i.e. glipizide) and meglitinides (i.e. nateglinide)
   D. GLP-1 receptor agonists (i.e. exenatide) and amylin analogs (i.e. pramlintide)

64. A patient states that he has the goal of getting his A1C to below 7% by the end of the year. He worries that having it high as it is now (7.9%) puts him at risk for complications. You notice his weight has been increasing. He admits that with his new job, he has not had time to work out at the gym and has been snacking a lot, due to stress. Which of the actions below would be a *best* next step with this patient?
   A. Discuss the increased risks of having a HbA1c level above 7%
   B. Ask open-ended questions that may help the patient identify some short–term goals that will help lower his A1c
   C. Lay out a daily schedule for the patient that facilitates his return to exercising, which will be sufficient to lower glucose levels without increasing his medication
   D. Explore why he eats when stressed and suggest some stress-reduction exercises that he can do at work.

65. Acute sensory neuropathy and chronic sensorimotor distal polyneuropathy (DPN) is characterized by severe burning pain in the lower extremities that is often worse at night. For treatment of these conditions, what is considered the key to effective management?
   A. Confirmation of diagnosis and ruling out other causes through neurologic testing
   B. Pain management with medication and referral to a pain management specialist
   C. Graded supervised aerobic exercise to safely improve circulation
   D. Blood glucose control and stabilization

66. Which of the following is an accurate association between celiac disease and diabetes?
   A. Celiac disease is associated with insulin resistance, and therefore has a greater prevalence among those with type 2 diabetes when compared to the general population.
   B. Because celiac disease is an immune-mediated disorder, there is a greater prevalence among those with type 1 diabetes when compared to the general population.
   C. Because wheat-free diets are naturally lower in carbohydrates, the celiac diet is a recommended meal plan option for those with type 2 diabetes, even without diagnosed celiac disease.
   D. Because celiac disease occurs with much greater frequency in the diabetic population (as compared to general population), screening for celiac is recommended for all persons with diabetes.

67. Which explanation best describes how steroid use *most* affects blood glucose?
   A. Steroid use induces insulin resistance and affects glucose metabolism, which is manifested especially in post-prandial glucose levels.
   B. Steroid use decreases the rate of insulin metabolism and therefore increases the risk for hypoglycemia.
   C. Steroid use increases insulin resistance and is specifically manifested in fasting glucose levels.
   D. Steroids suppress the immune system and deactivate a portion of both endogenous and exogenous insulin. Therefore, blood glucose typically rises with steroid use.

68. You call to follow up with your patient, who was diagnosed with diabetes six weeks ago. She admits that after she used all her blood glucose test strips, she quit checking her blood sugar because she has no insurance and they are too expensive for her very limited income. Which of the following resources would be *least* helpful to this patient?
    A. Partnership for Prescription Assistance (a national program sponsored by pharmaceutical research companies)
    B. A low-interest medical loan from her local bank
    C. The local or state health department low-income prescription program
    D. Needymeds.com (a non-profit organization that centralizes information and applications for pharmaceutical drug assistance programs)

69. The Diabetes Prevention Program demonstrated that progression from prediabetes to type 2 diabetes can be delayed or even prevented through lifestyle modifications and weight reduction. Based on the results of this large-scale study, what does the American Diabetes Association recommend as a target weight reduction for those with prediabetes?
    A. 10 to 20 pounds
    B. 7% of body weight
    C. Weight loss to within 10 pounds of ideal body weight
    D. Body mass index (BMI) of 22 or less

70. Which two risk factors have the strongest correlation with a patient's risk for development and progression of diabetic retinopathy?
    A. Type of diabetes and HbA1c
    B. Blood glucose control and blood pressure control
    C. Blood glucose variability and smoking status
    D. Blood pressure control and family history of eye disease

71. What is the recommended breakdown of macronutrients, according to the current American Diabetes Association Nutrition Recommendations (2013)?
    A. Approximately 70% of total calories should come carbohydrates, 20% from protein, and 10% from fat
    B. Approximately 45 to 55% of total calories should come carbohydrates, 25 to 40% from protein, and 15 to 20% from fat
    C. Approximately 35 to 40% of total calories should come carbohydrates, 20 to 30% from protein, and 30 to 35% from fat
    D. There is no specific mix of macronutrients recommended by the ADA. The best mix of macronutrients depends on individual circumstances

72. Which dietary strategy is the primary recommendation for those with prediabetes?
    A. A meal plan that focuses on moderate carbs, including carb monitoring/counting
    B. A low-carbohydrate diet (i.e. Atkins diet or similar)
    C. A calorie-reduced diet with reduced intake of dietary fat
    D. A low glycemic-index/glycemic-load diet

73. Which of the following food options would be the best example of an appropriate treatment option for a blood glucose level of 58 mg/dL?
    A. 8 oz. whole milk
    B. 15 grapes
    C. 2 Tbsp. peanut butter
    D. 2 Tbsp. peanut butter on a slice of bread

74. Lipohypertrophy is described as "thickened tumor-like swelling of the subcutaneous tissue or a mild swelling or lump under the skin at injection sites." When insulin is injected into these spots, insulin absorption is significantly decreased. What counsel should be given to a patient who exhibits signs of lipohypertrophy?

    A. Begin antibiotic therapy under the direction of a dermatologist to reduce the swelling

    B. Apply warm compresses twice daily until the swelling is significantly reduced

    C. Avoid injecting insulin into those areas until the swelling is gone; rotate injection sites to prevent recurrence

    D. These swollen masses must be removed surgically, but this can typically be done as an outpatient procedure in a dermatology office

75 You have a patient with type 1 diabetes (on MDI) who tells you that for religious reasons, he would like to fast one day each month (from after dinner until about 3 PM the next day – about 20 hours). Which response and action would be most appropriate?

    A. Discuss possible challenges and the best way to address them, such as more frequent monitoring, consideration of insulin pump therapy, and plan to address high or low blood sugars.

    B. Readdress the hazards of fasting with the patient, including hypoglycemia and DKA. Warn the patient that fasting is not advised for those with type 1 diabetes.

    C. Offer to explain the health concerns to the patient's pastor in hopes that an alternative arrangement can be made for the patient.

    D. Tell the patient that if he chooses to fast, he should take only half his basal insulin and no bolus insulin. For hypoglycemia, he should use a glucagon injection.

76. During a visit with your patient, a 68-year old man with type 2 diabetes, you discuss his physical activity goal that was set six months ago. His goal was to begin a walking program starting at 10 minutes per day and advance until he is walking 30 minutes per day at the six-month point. He rates his progress towards his goal at a "0" and says that he has not done anything since he set the goal at his visit six months ago. What is next *best* step to take with this patient?

    A. Suggest that he not dwell on this failed goal and focus on a different aspect of self management

    B. Offer the patient more time to work on his goal

    C. Discuss with the patient his motivations and barriers to achieving the goal

    D. Suggest that the goal be revised to begin with less time walking and increase the time at a slower rate

77. In a multidisciplinary team care approach to diabetes management, which of the individuals below is "central to the team," according to the National Standards for DSME/DSMS?

    A. The patient

    B. The diabetes educator

    C. The case manager

    D. The primary care physician

78. You are teaching a group class on diabetes and healthy meal planning. All four participants have provided an example of what they consider a healthy, well-balanced meal for someone who has diabetes. Which example would you site as the *best* example of an appropriate meal choice?
   A. A turkey and cheese, lettuce, and tomato sandwich with an apple, a small serving of baked chips, and a diet soda
   B. A bowl of chicken broth, pickle, sugar-free Jell-O, 2 celery sticks, water, and a multiple vitamin
   C. A medium chef salad with lettuce, eggs, cheese, chicken, celery, and Italian dressing, and a glass of water
   D. Whole-grain pasta (about 2 cups) with low-fat cream sauce, 1 slice of garlic bread, 1 cup of cooked green peas, and skim milk

79. Blood pressure readings for a pregnant patient (26 weeks' gestation) with gestational diabetes at her last three visits were as follows: 134/92, 144/90, and 142/96. She is already on a low-salt diet and says she follows it consistently. Which, if any, of the treatment options below would be appropriate for this patient?
   A. Methyldopa
   B. A low-dose of an ACE inhibitor (i.e. lisinopril)
   C. A low-to-moderate dose of a diuretic (i.e. furosemide)
   D. No medical treatment is necessary, as these levels are mostly within target for pregnancy. Reinforce lifestyle modification, including a low-salt diet and regular walking.

80. The prescribed meal plan for your patient is based on a 2000-calorie requirement. The number of calories coming from saturated fat should not exceed what amount?
   A. Calories from saturated for this patient should not exceed 40 calories per day.
   B. Calories from saturated fat for this patient should not exceed 140 to 200 calories per day.
   C. Saturated fat, in all persons with diabetes, should not exceed 200 mg per day, regardless of total calorie need.
   D. There is no recommendation for saturated fat, but total fat calories for this patient should not exceed 700 calories.

81. Mrs. M is a 65-year-old Hispanic female with type 2 diabetes and a diagnosis of congestive heart failure. At this time, she takes no medication for her diabetes, and states that she follows a fairly strict carb-consistent diet. Her A1c values have steadily increased over the past year and have now reached 8.4%. In addition, her serum creatinine has also been increasing and is now at 2.1 mg/dL. She states she is not willing to consider insulin at this time. Which medication would you recommend her provider prescribe for Mrs. M?
   A. Glucophage® (metformin)
   B. Actos® (pioglitazone)
   C. Lantus® insulin (insulin glargine)
   D. Januvia® (sitagliptin)

82. Which of the following statements below is a recent evidence-based practice recommendation and an example of translating research into practice?
   A. Low-carbohydrate diets are recommended for persons with type 2 diabetes because of results showing greater weight loss and improvements in lipid levels
   B. Unvaccinated adults with diabetes who are aged 19 through 59 years should receive hepatitis B vaccination
   C. Routine antioxidant supplementation, including vitamins A and C and carotene, is recommended for adults with type 2 diabetes.
   D. Glycemic goals for critical-care hospitalized patients with diabetes should not exceed 120 mg/dL and should not be less than 80 mg/dL.

83. A patient with uncontrolled type 2 diabetes, a sedentary lifestyle, and multiple co-morbidities tells you that she wishes to begin an exercise program to lose weight and improve her overall health. She states she wants to start slowly (walking and mild weight training), but eventually work up to where she can run a mile with her husband. Her co-morbidities include, "severe non-proliferative retinopathy" (according to ophthalmologist notes from 7 months ago), stage 2 renal disease with microalbuminuria, cardiac autonomic neuropathy, and peripheral neuropathy that is manifested by reduced sensation in her feet. Which of the following statements is most accurate and complete, regarding pre-exercise evaluation and referrals?
   A. Because the patient is starting slowly (i.e. walking and mild weight training), no referral or extensive pre-exercise physical evaluation is needed.
   B. The patient should receive an electrocardiogram stress test since she is currently sedentary. No other referrals are warranted at this time.
   C. This patient should be referred for an ECG stress test and a retinopathy exam. In addition, the provider should perform a thorough physical exam and the patient may need to modify the exercise regimen to prevent exacerbation of her complications.
   D. This patient should have referrals to ophthalmology, neurology, cardiology, nephrology, and possibly to an exercise physiologist. All team members will need to confer on this patient to devise the best activity regimen; it is likely that exercise will be contraindicated due to the extensive high-risk co-morbidities.

84. You have been asked to provide a 90-minute diabetes education activity at a senior center for six to twelve residents, all of who have diabetes. Group members will have different levels of pre-existing diabetes knowledge. Which instructional strategy below would be *most* appropriate? (Assume that you have access to or will be provided any equipment and furniture that may be needed and that you are equally comfortable with all strategies.)
   A. Conversation maps
   B. Computer/web-based DSME (you have access to six laptops)
   C. Providing printed diabetes materials to address a variety of topics; use activity time to go over what each publication addresses
   D. PowerPoint lecture addressing basic diabetes principles

85. Listed below are types of teaching strategies. Each has attributes and limitations. If you were choosing appropriate strategies based *solely* upon group size (from *individual* to *large group*), select the series that makes the most sense.
   A. Games, printed materials, demonstration, case studies
   B. Web-based activities, role-playing, group discussion, lecture
   C. Printed materials, lecture, demonstration, Web-based activities
   D. Games, lecture, printed material, group discussion

86. In speaking with a group of new inpatient nurses, you discuss the American Association of Clinical Endocrinologist (AACE) and American Diabetes Association (ADA) consensus statement (2009) recommendations of inpatient blood glucose targets. Which of the following statements accurately reflects those recommendations?
    A. Pre-meal BG target for non-critically ill patients: < 100 mg/dL
    B. Random BG target for non-critically ill patients: < 140 mg/dL
    C. Target (all times) BG for critically ill patients: 100 to 130 mg/dL
    D. Target (all times) BG for critically ill patients: 140 to 180 mg/dL

87. Your patient with type 2 diabetes is committed to exercising faithfully to both improve her glycemic control as well as lose weight. However, whenever she exercises beyond 30 minutes (at moderate intensity), her blood glucose drops below 80 mg/dL and she has to consume some type of sugary snack to bring it up. She is very discouraged that she is not able to lose weight due to having to supplement with extra sugar and calories when she exercises. Which of the following possible adjustments would be the best choice to make to the patient's regimen to prevent hypoglycemia and address her concern about weight loss?
    A. She might consume a small amount of fat-free fruit before the activity (i.e. half a glass of orange juice)
    B. She could omit her breakfast dose of repaglinide (Prandin®) on the mornings she will exercise
    C. She could skip her morning dose of metformin on mornings she will exercise
    D. She should not be concerned about the weight at this point as exercise has many other benefits, and she needs to treat low blood sugar

88. Your patient has had type 2 diabetes for the past twelve years. He controls his diabetes with diet, exercise, and oral medication. Similarly, he watches his fat intake because of occasional borderline LDL (currently WNL). His last three HbA1c labs were all less than 7%. He has no apparent co-morbidities. According to the American Diabetes Association Standards of Practice (2013), which of the following screenings is not indicated *annually* for this patient?
    A. HbA1c
    B. Comprehensive foot exam
    C. Dilated eye exam
    D. Fasting lipid profile

89. Your patient arrives late for his appointment. You notice that his HbA1c is higher and that his adherence to self-care skills (specifically monitoring, exercising and taking medication) has decreased since his last visit 6 months ago. When you ask, "Over the last month or so, have you lost interest in doing things that usually bring you pleasure?" He replies, "Yes, I have to admit that I have." What implication does this have and what should your response be?

    A. His answer suggests that the patient is in a "slump" (or "burnout"), which many people with diabetes experience. Assure him it is normal and encourage him to think back to how he felt when he was faithfully performing self-care behaviors.

    B. His answer is expected, for when a person neglects self-care behaviors, it negatively affects glucose levels, which then decreases one's ability to participate in pleasurable activities. Discuss this cycle with the patient and encourage him to be more diligent with his monitoring, exercise, and medication.

    C. The patient's answer suggests that he may be experiencing diabetes-related anxiety. Stress, the body's response to the anxiety, is manifested in his increased HbA1c and neglect of self-care activities. Discuss ways to reduce anxiety and stress, such as medication or breathing exercises.

    D. His response is a strong indicator of depression. Encourage the patient to meet with a mental health professional; then make the referral and offer to help schedule the appointment. Follow up with the patient by phone to ensure that he attended the appointment and schedule a follow-up visit for diabetes care in one month.

90. You are meeting with your patient who has type 2 diabetes and is pregnant (26 weeks). She reports that her fasting and post-prandial blood glucose values have been within the target range and that she is taking insulin before each meal as advised. However, she also reports that almost every day of the last two weeks, she has had a small-to-moderate amount of ketones in her urine. Of the options below, which management plan would best address this problem?

    A. As long as ketones are not consistently large and her blood glucose values are within range, there is no need to adjust her regimen at this time.

    B. The patient's bedtime long-acting insulin dose should be increased to eliminate the ketones.

    C. Since ketones are a byproduct of the breakdown of fat, the patient should increase the amount of fat eaten throughout the day so that she will gain weight instead of lose it.

    D. The patient should add a substantial snack at bedtime, coupled with a dose of prandial insulin to cover the snack.

91. Which of the following statements concerning treatment for peripheral arterial disease (PAD) is *true*?

    A. Reduction of blood pressure (by about 10/5 mmHg) has been shown to reduce the risk of amputation in PAD by 30%.

    B. Control of blood glucose at an HbA1c of 7% or lower has been shown to significantly slow the progression of existing PAD.

    C. Lipid lowering has been associated with nearly 40% reduction in new or worsening symptoms of PAD.

    D. Casual (unsupervised) exercise programs have been shown to have excellent benefits for those with PAD, including reduction of PAD symptoms, increased circulation, and improved balance.

92. Despite attending all classes as well as one-on-one visits with the educator, a patient performs only the bare minimum self-care skills. Beyond basic survival skills education, he has not been receptive to any additional information about his diabetes. Which explanation below is the most likely, and what is the logical course of action for the educator?
    A. He did not fully understand the information in the classes; he would likely benefit from a review of the self-management material.
    B. His personality is more introspective; he likely uses the "problem-focused coping style." This patient should be presented with printed information that he can process privately and provided with contact information, should he need help.
    C. The patient is likely experiencing the "depression & frustration" emotional stage of a chronic disease. The educator should emphasize positive changes and accomplishments, but recognize the sense of loss that comes with facing a lifetime disease.
    D. The patient's actions represent an "avoidant coping style," commonly associated with emotional discomfort. The educator should initiate a frank, honest discussion on what he is feeling, including validating his feelings. "Pushing" additional, more "in-depth" diabetes education at this point is not helpful.

93. Jeff is a 26 year old with type 1 diabetes; he wears an insulin pump. He reports that he has noticed a pattern of hypoglycemia two to three hours after lunch and dinner. When asked, he states that before meals, and even after breakfast, he seems to have no problem. Which of the following pump setting changes would you recommend?
    A. Reducing his basal rate by 10% between lunch and bedtime
    B. Changing his insulin-to-carb ratio from 10 to 12 for lunch and dinner only
    C. Modifying his correction/sensitivity factor to give less insulin
    D. Changing insulin-to-carb ratio from 10 to 8 for lunch and dinner only

94. Assuming each of the patients below are currently consuming an average amount of daily protein (about 0.8 to 1.0 g/kg body wt. /day), which of the patients may need to *reduce* his or her daily protein intake?
    A. A pregnant woman, normal weight, in second trimester
    B. A 60-year-old male with stage 4 kidney disease, normal BMI
    C. A female (type 2) with a slow-healing lower-extremity wound
    D. None of the above should be switched to a low-protein diet

95. Which of the following behavioral objectives below is an example of an *immediate outcome*?
    A. Demonstrating proper technique for self monitoring blood glucose
    B. Reducing the number of missed doses of medication
    C. Improving HDL to target level
    D. Being 100% compliant on all recommended screenings

96. Some dietary supplements are packaged in containers with a "USP-verified mark". What is the role of the US Pharmacopoeia (USP) and thus indicated by this label?
    A. To verify that the products listed on the label are accurate and pure
    B. To market herbal products that have been FDA approved
    C. To verify that the clinical claims made by the products are accurate
    D. To ensure that herbal supplements will not interact with other medications

97. Which of the following accurately describes the policy on disposing of sharps, such as insulin syringes, lancets, and infusion set needles?
   A. Used sharps should only ever be put into official biohazard (sharps) containers, which can be purchased at a pharmacy.
   B. It is okay to put sharps in a hard plastic container (such as a laundry detergent bottle) and when full, tape the lid and throw it away in the regular garbage.
   C. Sharps may be put in a hard, non-permeable container, but should be taken to the pharmacy for final disposal, and never put in the regular garbage collection.
   D. Since medical waste disposal laws vary from state to state, patients and educators need to determine specific policy for their areas.

98. Your patient takes basal insulin with a sulfonylurea. You meet with him to consider adjustment to his current regimen, at the patient's request. His recent A1c was 8.9%. At the appointment, he states that he is not sure where the problem lies, and he expresses frustration that his insurance will only cover 4 bottles of test strips (200 test strips) every two months. Which self-monitoring regimen below would be the *most* appropriate for this patient?
   A. Right before and two hours after a single meal day, rotating the meal. Do this for two to three weeks and then bring in results.
   B. Fasting morning monitoring every morning and then again just before bed every night, for one month.
   C. Because this patient takes insulin, he needs to test before each meal, every day, indefinitely.
   D. Due to his limitation on test strips, he should save them for when he feels his blood glucose may be high or low, and rely on other records, such as food and exercise logs to pinpoint the problem.

99. After exhausting other medical options, a patient's physician prescribes insulin for his hospitalized patient, and recommends the regimen be continued at home after discharge. The patient has a very limited income as well as very poor eyesight; the patient is unable to drive to follow-up visits or to pick up prescriptions at the pharmacy. Which healthcare (hospital staff) team member should you most likely consult to assist the patient?
   A. Pharmacist
   B. Registered dietitian
   C. Inpatient social worker
   D. Ordering physician

100. What is the ultimate goal of diabetes self-management education and support?
   A. Optimal glycemic control
   B. Imparting knowledge and skills needed to make important lifestyle (behavioral) changes
   C. Reduction of diabetes-related complications
   D. Reduced incidence, cost, and effects of diabetes through improved prevention, diagnosis, and management

101. Which of the following is a difference between medication administration using a disposable insulin pen device to inject insulin and a pen device to inject a GLP-1 analog medication, such as exenatide (Byetta®)?
   A. Insulin pen devices require a new pen needle each time, but with GLP-1 receptor agonist pen devices, the same needle can be used repeatedly.
   B. Insulin injections require site rotation, but GLP-1 receptor agonist injections can be given in the same spot since they are typically given less frequently.
   C. When using an insulin pen device, the patient should prime the pen (perform an "air shot") before each use, whereas with a GLP-1 agonist medication, the priming is only done as part of new pen setup (before first use of each pen).
   D. GLP-1 agonist medication must be kept refrigerated until immediately before use, whereas an in-use insulin pen may be kept at room temperature until the use limit (i.e. 28 days for insulin aspart or insulin glargine).

102. Which of the choices below is the *best* example of a behavioral goal/objective that is *specific*?
   A. "Decrease intake of regular soda from three cans to one can per day by Dec. 1"
   B. "Decrease the risk for diabetes-related cardiovascular complications by 25%"
   C. "Improve glycemic control by the next diabetes care visit"
   D. "Improve overall health by eating better, moving more, and getting better rest"

103. Which of the following methods is *not* recommended as an effective way to obtain information on tracking behavioral objectives?
   A. Group classes
   B. Email messaging
   C. Phone consultation
   D. Any of the above are legitimate ways to track patient progress of behavioral goals

104. Your patient takes insulin glargine (Lantus®) and has a treat-to-target self-adjustment scale, with a fasting morning glucose target of ≤120 mg/dL. It has been three months since his last visit. Since his last visit, his basal insulin dose has been self-increased by 18 units (to 48 units QHS). Today, his BG meter shows that his fasting glucose levels are still usually above target, sometimes within target, with an occasional hypoglycemic reading. Most bedtime glucose readings are well above target. You also notice that his weight has increased by 4 kg (about 9 pounds) since his last visit. What is the most likely explanation for these findings?
   A. The patient requires additional basal insulin since most of his fasting morning readings are still above target. He should increase his dose according to the algorithm.
   B. He requires additional basal insulin, but because he is taking more than 40 units, he may benefit by having a split dose (i.e. 25 units at night and 25 units at bedtime).
   C. Because he has some low readings (although few), he should decrease the dose and add bolus (mealtime) insulin during the day.
   D. As evidenced by his weight gain and continued high readings, the patient is likely overeating. Help the patient evaluate current eating patterns and make adjustments.

- 154 -

105. Your patient, a 24-year old with type 1 diabetes for three years, manages his diabetes with multiple daily injections of basal and rapid-acting insulin. He reports a trend of high morning blood sugars and hypoglycemia just before meals during the day. The patient agrees to wear a continuous glucose-monitoring sensor (CGMS) for three days. Upon examination of the report, you notice two occurrences where the patient's blood glucose dropped below 60 mg/dL overnight. On the one night when this did not occur, fasting morning blood sugars were within target range. What is the likely explanation for what this patient is experiencing?
   A. Somogyi phenomenon
   B. Dawn phenomenon
   C. Inappropriate nutrient balance at night (needs more protein)
   D. Fluctuations in the honeymoon period

The following patient case applies to the next six questions:

> B. Jones, a 78-year old African-American male, newly diagnosed with type 2 diabetes, is accompanied by his daughter for his initial DSME assessment visit. He admits that he has poor eyesight (at least close-up) and sometimes forgets things. He states that he is willing to learn about his diabetes and is willing to make some minor changes in his lifestyle if it will help him have more energy to play golf and play with his grandchildren. He does not do much cooking (he leaves that to his daughter or eats out); presently he walks for 15 minutes each weekday and plays 9 holes of golf every weekend. His BMI is 25, BP is within normal limits and A1c at this time is 8.2%. He states that has no known diabetes-related complications; his daughter confirms this and his patient medical record lists none either.

106. Based on his statements, Mr. Jones most fits which transtheoretical model stage of change?
   A. Precontemplation
   B. Contemplation
   C. Action
   D. Maintenance

107. Which of the following would be an appropriate behavioral objective (both in terms of the goal itself and how it is stated) for Mr. Jones?
   A. "I will choose items from the restaurant menu that fit with my healthy eating plan, including vegetables, low-fat meat, and 3 servings of carbohydrates."
   B. "I will understand the reasons that I need to monitor my blood sugar."
   C. "I will know the difference between my diabetes medications."
   D. "By modifying eating patterns, taking medication, and increasing frequency of self-monitoring, my A1c will be within less than 8% within six months."

108. Which question below is the best example of an appropriate patient empowerment question you might ask Mr. Jones?
   A. "You do not want to end up on dialysis, do you?"
   B. "What do you think your A1c should be?"
   C. "What effect do you think changes such as taking your medication and eating better might have on your daily life?"
   D. "I think that we need to set a goal for you to lose some weight. Ten pounds would put you closer to a normal BMI. How does that sound to you?"

109. Which of the following is an example of an instructional method that would be *least* appropriate for Mr. Jones?
   A. Group discussion on choosing healthy food options at a restaurant
   B. One-on-one, hands-on BG meter training
   C. Role-playing on how Mr. Jones would react if he accidentally took a double dose of his diabetes medication
   D. Printed material (package insert) from manufacturer regarding the side effects of the medications

110. Which of the following options below is the *best* example of an appropriate "S.M.A.R.T." (specific, measurable, attainable, realistic, timely) behavioral goal for Mr. Jones?
   A. Lose ten pounds by October 31 (3 months) by increasing walking to 25 minutes per day and limiting second helpings to just vegetables.
   B. Reduce A1c to 6% by October 31 (3 months) by checking blood glucose twice daily and starting insulin.
   C. Improving diabetes and overall health by doing the things Mr. Jones learned in the diabetes class.
   D. Take good care of himself for the rest of his life by eating better, taking medicine consistently, checking blood sugar, getting good rest, checking feet daily, and keeping all medical appointments.

111. Mr. Jones's provider has prescribed him Januvia® (sitagliptin) QD and a sulfonylurea BID, with a note in the chart to possibly initiate insulin if the patient's A1c is not less than 8% in six months. Which of the following items is *least* important in the initial education plan for this patient?
   A. How to use an insulin pen
   B. Preventing, recognizing, and treating hypoglycemia
   C. Making appropriate food choices
   D. Prevention of diabetes-related complications

112. What is the *greatest* risk for persons with small-nerve-fiber neuropathy (a subcategory of chronic sensorimotor distal neuropathy)?
   A. Injury from falls due to Charcot foot syndrome
   B. Decrease in overall wellness due to limited mobility
   C. Risk for sudden cardiac death due to cardiac denervation
   D. Foot ulceration and subsequent gangrene and amputation

113. Regarding communication among all members of a patient's healthcare team, which of the following statements is *true*, according to the National Standards for Diabetes Self-management and Support (2013)?
   A. Because of HIPAA restrictions, providers and educators are limited in sharing patients' health information with team members without permission from the patients.
   B. Sharing information among healthcare team members increases the likelihood that all the members will work in collaboration.
   C. Patients report greater satisfaction when their information is shared among team members, and it saves them the time of having to have repeat assessments.
   D. Communicating with members of a patient's healthcare team under recent guidelines has resulted in additional cost in terms of time, money, and work burden.

114 In the last few years, professional diabetes organizations including the ADA have adopted the A1c test as a diagnostic tool. In order for a valid diagnosis to be made using the HbA1c of ≥ 6.5%, which of the following stipulations or qualifiers must also be present?
   A. HbA1c must be accompanied by a fasting glucose test of over 126 mg/dL
   B. The patient must also have symptoms of hyperglycemia
   C. The patient must also have at least one episode of random plasma glucose >180 mg/dL
   D. HbA1c test must be NGSP-certified and standardized to the Diabetes Complications and Control Trial (DCCT); repeat test is recommended.

115. You receive the lab results for your next patient and see the HbA1c is 9.6%. When the patient enters the room, she tells you that she forgot her meter but brought her log book. You see that for the past two months, she has not missed a single pre-meal or bedtime blood glucose test. All numbers are within target range. What is the most likely explanation for the discrepancy?
   A. The patient likely has some type of anemia or hemoglobinopathy which results in her HbA1c not closely correlating with actual average estimated glucose.
   B. The patient likely had a brand of BG meter that is inaccurate.
   C. The patient is likely making up blood glucose values
   D. The patient is probably using improper testing technique.

116. Which of the following dietary interventions has *not* been shown to be an effective weight-loss strategy?
   A. Four to 5 small meals/snacks throughout the day
   B. Omitting breakfast to reduce total daily caloric intake
   C. Emphasis on portion control
   D. Meal replacements (such as liquid meals or pre-packaged weight loss meals)

117. What is the *first* treatment priority for a person experiencing a hyperosmolar hyperglycemic state (HHS)?
   A. Decrease blood glucose by infusing insulin
   B. Rehydrate by providing adequate intravenous fluids
   C. Correct electrolyte imbalances by monitoring and providing supplementation when needed
   D. Address the background infection that precipitates the HHS

118. Which of the following statements regarding HbA1c is *accurate*, in relation to persons with diabetes?
   A. Regardless of age or other factors, an HbA1c greater than 7% represents a medically unacceptable risk.
   B. HbA1c was recently adopted by the American Diabetes Association as a diagnostic tool for diabetes because there is almost no variation among race, gender, or age and it remains largely unaffected by other medical conditions.
   C. Screening for diabetes by using the HbA1c has been shown to identify more cases of previously undiagnosed diabetes than either the fasting plasma glucose or the 2-hour glucose tolerance test.
   D. The ADA recommends that the HbA1c test should be performed at least twice annually, and more often in some cases.

119. To determine a patient's level of mastery of self-care skills such as insulin administration, which of the following evaluation methods should be used?
  A. Return demonstration
  B. Ask the patient to explain the process
  C. Ask the patient to verbally acknowledge understanding of the skill
  D. Completion of a short post test (which can be quantified/scored)

120. Which statement regarding dental disease and diabetes is *false*?
  A. Treatment of periodontal disease has been shown to reduce HbA1c levels
  B. Children with diabetes have significantly more dental caries than their non-diabetic counterparts.
  C. Elevated glucose increases the frequency, progression, and severity of periodontal disease.
  D. Medication such as diuretics and antidepressants may contribute to tooth decay and periodontal disease.

121. Which of the following lab findings is *most* closely associated with hypertriglyceridemia?
  A. High HDL
  B. Elevated fasting plasma glucose
  C. Low HDL
  D. Small-sized LDL-C particles

122. Which of the following is the primary role of the diabetes educator regarding depression and diabetes?
  A. Using a reliable, valid tool to diagnose patients who exhibit symptoms
  B. Teaching patients depression prevention strategies, including stress management techniques
  C. Screening patients and assisting them in getting access to care from a mental health professional
  D. Conferring with the mental health professional to know how to appropriately counsel depressed patients on diabetes self care

123. Which stage of diabetic retinopathy is characterized by neovascularization (new vessel growth) and/or vitreous or preretinal hemorrhage?
  A. Proliferative diabetic retinopathy
  B. Severe nonproliferative diabetic retinopathy
  C. Moderate nonproliferative diabetic retinopathy
  D. Mild nonproliferative diabetic retinopathy

124. For hospitalized patients with diabetes, discharge planning, including appropriate diabetes education (i.e. "survival skills" education) should begin when?
  A. As soon as the patient is admitted
  B. As soon as the provider has written the discharge order
  C. As soon as the patient stated that he or she is ready for instruction
  D. As soon as the appropriate diabetes treatment plan (i.e. diet recommendations, medications, SMBG schedule and targets) has been decided

125. Which electrolyte level, frequently masked and appearing as normal, can be life threatening if not immediately corrected in diabetic ketoacidosis (DKA)?
   A. Potassium
   B. Phosphate
   C. Sodium bicarbonate
   D. Sodium

126. Which of the follow statements is true regarding preconception care and diabetes?
   A. Only about half of all female patients of childbearing age with diabetes receive preconception counseling.
   B. Preconception care should include weight management as the first priority so that those women who become pregnant are as close to ideal body weight as possible.
   C. The rate of congenital malformations for diabetic women whose HbA1c is less than 7% prior to and at conception is similar to rates for women without diabetes.
   D. An important part of preconception counseling may be to initiate lipid management medication (such as a statin), since lipid levels tend to increase during the first part of pregnancy.

127. At a visit last month, your patient committed to quit smoking. When you call to see how he is doing (four weeks later), he admits that he has had two relapses, but then "re-committed" to stop smoking each time. He asks if you have any tips to help him avoid these relapses. Which suggestion below is *not* a recommended relapse prevention strategy?
   A. Be aware of risky behavior or situations that may lead to a relapse and try to avoid them
   B. Have a plan to combat negative thoughts or temptations
   C. Employ stress management techniques, such as cognitive reframing, turning to a support person, or others that the patient has used to help manage stress
   D. Acknowledge and repeat the mantra that the bad behavior is gone and will not come back (i.e. "I am not a smoker; I do not want or need to smoke").

128. Hypoglycemia unawareness is the decrease or absence of the typical counterregulatory responses to low blood glucose. Which of the following options is the *primary* recommendation for addressing this phenomenon?
   A. More frequent blood glucose monitoring, including use of continuous glucose monitoring
   B. Less stringent glucose targets, at least for several weeks
   C. More stringent blood glucose control to restore autonomic responses to hypoglycemia
   D. Increased precautions, including cessation of driving and limits on high-risk activity

129. You are instructing insulin-requiring patients on how to treat hypoglycemia. To treat hypoglycemia that occurs immediately before a meal, which of the following is the best course of action?
   A. Skip your insulin because your blood sugar is already too low. If the glucose is normal or high before the next meal, then you may take the recommended dose at that time.
   B. Eat your meal now but take your dose of mealtime insulin about an hour later.
   C. Treat the blood sugar as you would any low blood sugar, and then once it is in the normal range, take your regular dose of insulin and eat your regular meal.
   D. Take the insulin right away, then prepare the meal and eat as you normally would.

130. Your patient comes in for a return visit one month after starting basal bolus insulin therapy. She tells you that she will have to stop taking half of her insulin because her insurance does not pay for Apidra® insulin, only Lantus®, and she cannot afford to pay out of pocket for it. Assuming that there may be other insulin brands in this class that her insurance does cover, which of the following insulins below would be the most appropriate replacement for Apidra® that you might suggest to this patient's provider?
    A. NPH/regular (Novolin 70/30®)
    B. Insulin detemir (Levemir®)
    C. NPH insulin (Humulin-N®)
    D. Insulin lispro (Humalog®)

131. Which of the following HbA1c targets would be *most* appropriate for a 69-year-old woman with long-standing type 1 diabetes who has cardiovascular disease, advanced kidney disease, retinopathy, and autonomic neuropathy?
    A. < 9.5%
    B. < 8%
    C. < 7%
    D. < 6.5%

132. According to the recently published ADA Nutrition Therapy Recommendations (2013), which of the following statements regarding outcomes of low-carbohydrate diets is *true*?
    A. The glycemic effects of low-carb diets is mixed, therefore, no definite conclusions can be drawn regarding the effects of low carb diets on HbA1c
    B. Low-carb diets were found to raise LDL and triglyceride levels in most studies
    C. Studies suggest that low-carb diets are effective because retention with these diets is high
    D. Low-carb diets are the safest option for a patient with renal disease

133. Which of the following is the *least* likely to result in low blood glucose?
    A. Decreased food intake
    B. Increased insulin
    C. Increased level of stress
    D. Increased intake of alcohol without carbohydrates

134. A member of the DSME class group asks a specific question about food choices during session 1. You typically address healthy eating in session 2. What is the *best* way to handle the situation?
    A. In order to capitalize on the apparent interest, abandon the present order of classes. Talk about food today and discuss session 1 material next time.
    B. Take a few minutes to briefly answer the question; acknowledge that many in the group likely have questions about food, and promise that this will be addressed in greater detail as part of the next session.
    C. Tell the client that if he will be patient and remember his question for next session, you will promise to address it first thing.
    D. Politely explain that there is a specific order in which the information needs to be presented to make the most sense. Ask him to limit his questions to the topic at hand but let him know that he may ask you one on one after class if he needs an immediate answer.

135. A patient tells you that she is very worried about "dropping too low" at night and therefore eats a bowl of ice cream every night and only takes a half dose of her nighttime basal insulin. Because this results in high fasting AM blood sugars, she has quit testing in the morning, because she is not willing to increase her basal insulin anyway. What mental health issue does this patient exhibit?
- A. Depression
- B. Eating disorder
- C. Denial
- D. Anxiety

136. Which of the following nutrition modifications is *not* recommended for patients who suffer from gastroparesis?
- A. Increased dietary fiber
- B. Frequent small meals
- C. Decreased dietary fat
- D. Soft (i.e. over-cooked) or liquid foods

137. Which of the following labs require the patient to fast (minimum 8-hour fast)?
- A. Lipid profile
- B. HbA1c
- C. Microalbumin
- D. ALT/AST

138. Why does the American Diabetes Association recommend the "development of standardized procedures for documentation, training health professionals to document appropriately, and the use of structured standardized forms based on current practice guidelines" in the National Standards for Diabetes Self Management & Support (2013)?
- A. Such documentation practices and attributes are required by TJC (The Joint Commission)
- B. Such documentation practices and attributes have been shown to improve documentation and may ultimately improve quality of care
- C. Such documentation practices and attributes will facilitate smoother clinic operations and reduce administrative costs
- D. Such documentation practices and attributes assist in the reimbursement process and are preferred by most insurance carriers

139. Which statement below is characteristic of a "patient empowerment" approach to DSME/DSMS, as opposed to more traditional behavioral theories?
- A. Patients must rely only on themselves to deal with the challenges of a chronic disease, such as diabetes.
- B. Patients learn from their own experiences and from observing the experiences of those around them.
- C. The choices that have the greatest effect on diabetes outcomes are made by patients, not by healthcare professionals.
- D. A patient's perception of how the community/society views a behavior will have a great impact on his or her intentions to adapt it.

140. A new patient reports that she is not sure what type of diabetes she has because no one has ever given her a clear answer. She is 46 years old and Caucasian, with a BMI of 20. She states that she has always been thin and active, and that no one in her family has diabetes that she knows of. With the exception of her father, who has rheumatoid arthritis and psoriasis, her family history is unremarkable. She was diagnosed with diabetes two years ago and claims she is able to keep her blood sugars in the normal range with a careful low-carb diet. When you check her labs, you see that her last A1c was 6.4%, and her C-peptide level was on the low end of normal. Labs are also positive for GAD and islet-cell antibodies. What type of diabetes does this patient *most* likely have?

    A. Type 2 diabetes
    B. Type 1 diabetes
    C. Latent autoimmune diabetes of adulthood (LADA)
    D. Maturity-onset diabetes in the young

The next 2 questions relate to the nutrition label.

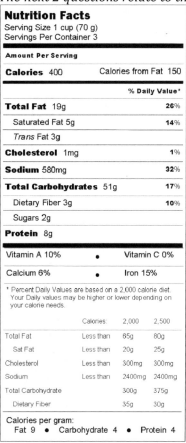

141. Your patient states that he eats about half the package of this product at one time. What is the approximate total amount of carbohydrates your patient consumes of this product?

    A. 25 g
    B. 51 g
    C. 75 g
    D. 102 g

142. The patient claims this is an ideal food for him. He says he is not worried about counting his carbs for this food because on the package it says the food is listed as a low-glycemic index food. Also, the label tells him that the sugars are pretty low and so based on that alone, this food is a good choice. Finally, the fiber is high, which means he doesn't need to count some of the carbohydrates. Which of the following conclusions below is *not* correct in this situation?
    A. The amount of fiber in this food is not high enough to discount from total carbohydrates.
    B. The total sugar is not important because the starches rapidly convert to glucose as well.
    C. Even though the food may be a low glycemic index food, moderation and tracking of all carbs is still needed.
    D. The patient is correct. The combination of low sugar, low glycemic index, and high fiber make this an ideal food choice, in any amount.

143. Which of the following diabetes medications should not be omitted for a patient who is fasting in preparation for surgery?
    A. Metformin
    B. Sulfonylurea
    C. Short-acting insulin
    D. Long-acting (basal) insulin

144. Which of the following foot care recommendations is *not* appropriate for a person with diabetes, assuming there are no physical limitations, severe neuropathy, or lower extremity injuries or infections?
    A. If foot odor is noticed, soak feet in a warm Epsom salt bath for 15 to 20 min. per day.
    B. If you notice dry skin, moisturize the area daily with lotion, except between the toes.
    C. Wash your feet frequently. Pat skin dry and dry between the toes thoroughly.
    D. If toenails are long enough to bump the inside of the shoe, trim straight across and file any sharp corners.

145. According to the 2013 ADA Standards of Care, what is the recommended maximum blood pressure target for most adults with diabetes who are being treated for hypertension?
    A. 120/80 mmHg
    B. 130/90 mmHg
    C. 120/90 mmHg
    D. 140/80 mmHg

146. Using the AADE7 Self-care Behaviors Goal Sheet, you and a patient are working on individualizing self-care behavior goals. You document that he has checked the box saying, "make better food choices" under the "Healthy Eating" category. Which of the following statements below is the best example of individualization of this goal?
    A. Make better food choices to reduce A1c to less than 7.5%
    B. Make better food choices over the next 6 months (by October 31)
    C. Switch to diet soda and sugar-free ice cream
    D. Report to educator each Monday on previous week's food choices

147. Which of these statements regarding obstructive sleep apnea is *not* accurate?
    A. Treatment of sleep apnea has been proven to significantly improve blood pressure control.
    B. Treatment of sleep apnea has been conclusively proven to improve glycemic control.
    C. Treatment of sleep apnea has been shown conclusively to improve quality of life.
    D. Persons who are obese are four to ten times more likely to have obstructive sleep apnea.

148. Which of the following is *not* a standard recommendation for those with mild-to-moderate chronic kidney disease (stages 1 through 4)?
   A. Restricting foods high in vitamin K (some leafy green vegetables)
   B. Good glycemic control (as tight as can be achieved without hypoglycemia)
   C. Blood pressure management through the use of an ACE inhibitor or ARB medication
   D. Abstaining from use of nonsteroidal anti-inflammatory drugs (NSAIDs)

149. Eating disorders are more common in those with diabetes than in the general population, and are more prevalent in women. Recent studies have been focused on women with type 1 diabetes who restrict insulin in order to avoid weight gain. Which of the following statements is *not* a finding of these studies?
   A. Withholding insulin to prevent weight gain is associated with problems in other diabetes self-care areas.
   B. Withholding insulin to prevent weight gain is associated with higher levels of diabetes-specific stress.
   C. Those women who withheld insulin to prevent weight gain have higher mortality risk, which correlates with the frequency of withholding the insulin.
   D. Those women who have had diabetes for shorter duration are more likely to restrict insulin than those who have had diabetes for longer duration

150. The FDA has approved six nonnutritive sweeteners for use in moderation: acesulfame-K, aspartame, Neotame, saccharin, sucralose, and Stevia. Which of these should be *avoided* by women who are pregnant or breastfeeding?
   A. Aspartame
   B. Saccharin
   C. Neotame
   D. All have been shown to be safe, even for pregnant or breastfeeding women

151. Which of the following patient attributes (skills/experiences) is *not* considered a prerequisite for continuous subcutaneous insulin infusion (i.e. insulin pump) therapy?
   A. Patient must have a diagnosis of type 1 diabetes
   B. Patient must be proficient at counting carbohydrates
   C. Patient should have previous experience on multiple daily injection (MDI) therapy
   D. Patient exhibits a pattern of consistent, frequent blood glucose monitoring

152. Which of the following reasons below is *not* listed as a rationale for documentation of patient encounters (including assessment, education plan and outcomes) under Standard 7 (Individualization) of the ADA National Standards for Diabetes Self Management & Support (2013)?
   A. Documentation provides proof of services rendered by the educator, and can be used to verify practice hours for certification renewal
   B. Documentation is used to guide the education process
   C. Documentation provides evidence of communication among instructional staff and other members of the participant's health care team
   D. Documentation prevents duplication of services

153. In a group class on nutrition, you show a sample breakfast menu and ask participants to modify the meals to measure about 60 grams of carbohydrate. One patient shares her modified menu: 1 scrambled egg, 2 oz. ham, 2 pieces of wheat toast, ½ large grapefruit, 1 cup skim milk. Which evaluation below best describes this meal?
   A. The meal has significantly too few grams of carbohydrates
   B. The meal has approximately 60 grams of carbohydrate
   C. The meal has significantly too many carbohydrates
   D. It is impossible to estimate the number of carbohydrates without seeing the grapefruit and the type of bread

154. For those who choose to consume alcoholic beverages, what guidelines do the American Diabetes Association provide in the Diabetes Standards of Care (2013)?
   A. One drink per day or less for adult women and two drinks per day or less for adult men is what is recommended for those who use alcohol.
   B. Two drinks per day or less for adult women and three drinks per day or less for adult men; abstaining from "hard liquor" is recommended.
   C. Persons with diabetes should not consume alcohol due to the increased risk for hypoglycemia.
   D. Persons with diabetes may consume alcohol without restriction as long as they account for carbohydrates and plan accordingly.

155. What is the blood pressure threshold at which patients with diabetes should be advised on lifestyle changes to reduce blood pressure?
   A. ≥150/90 mmHg
   B. ≥140/80 mmHg
   C. ≥130/80 mmHg
   D. >120/80 mmHg

156. Your patient is beginning a physical activity regimen, to include moderate intensity exercise 5 days a week for 30 minutes each day. He wants to know how to tell if he is exercising at the right intensity. From previous encounters with the patient, you are aware that he has some literacy/numeracy challenges, and so you decide to suggest the original "Rating of Perceived Exertion" (RPE). How would you explain this intensity guide to your patient?
   A. The RPE lets you estimate how intense your physical activity is by counting the number of breaths per minute and comparing it to the number at rest. Moderate/vigorous-intensity is equal to an increase of two to four breaths per minute.
   B. The RPE estimates intensity by how easy it is to have a conversation during the activity. For moderate/vigorous-intensity, you should be breathing harder but still be able to talk while performing the activity. If you are breathing too heavily to talk, then the activity is too intense.
   C. The RPE has you estimate the intensity of your activity based on how much your heart rate has increased (from resting). For every 10 beats per minute, you go up one number in the scale. You should be between a "5" and "8" (or 50 to 80 bpm increase) for moderate/vigorous-intensity activity.
   D. The RPE helps you estimate the intensity of your activity by focusing on how tired you feel and how difficult the activity seems. It uses a scale of 6 ("extremely light") to 20 ("beyond extremely hard" or "maximal exertion"). Moderate/vigorous-intensity activity is about 12 to 16 ("somewhat hard" to "hard") on the scale.

157. Your patient, who has just been prescribed two oral medications for type 2 diabetes, also takes many other medications for chronic conditions, including Crohn's disease, COPD, hypertension, anemia, and vitamin deficiencies. She is very concerned about medication dose timing, contraindications, and side effects; she requests an educational appointment to address her concerns. Which team member would be the best professional to meet with this patient?
   A. The doctor(s) who originally prescribed each medication
   B. A mental health professional to help her with anxiety
   C. The pharmacist assigned to the patient's healthcare team
   D. The registered dietitian, who is also a certified diabetes educator

158. Which of the following behavioral goals is *measurable*?
   A. "Improve diabetes control by managing my portion size"
   B. "Increase cardiovascular endurance by January 1"
   C. "Run 20 minutes at least three times per week"
   D. "Minimize the risk of diabetic eye disease by keeping my ophthalmology appointments"

159. Which of the following elements is *not* part of the standard "exercise prescription"?
   A. Commencement (when will the patient begin the activity program)
   B. Intensity (how difficult and challenging should the activity be)
   C. Frequency (how often with the activity be performed)
   D. Duration (how long will the activity last for each session)

160. All of the following suggestions below are appropriate strategies to address financial barriers associated with self-monitoring of blood glucose (SMBG), except one. Which suggestion is *not* a recommended cost-cutting strategy?
   A. Obtain a generic meter with corresponding test strips from a department store such as Wal-Mart, where test strips are only about half the cost.
   B. If possible, back-date the meter so that it will accept recently-expired test strips.
   C. Select a monitoring schedule/strategy that conserves test strips but still provides information to recognize trends.
   D. Regardless of the meter the clinic prefers, contact the insurance carrier to determine which meter/strips is preferred and therefore least expensive to the patient.

161. How frequently should most patients with diabetes receive a pneumonia vaccine (as recommended by the American Diabetes Association, 2013) in order to reduce the risks associated with pneumonia?
   A. One time for those over age 2, then a one-time revaccination for those age 65 or older
   B. Every year
   C. Every five years, unless the person has had pneumonia, and then vaccination is unnecessary
   D. Every ten years until age 80, at which time revaccination is not recommended

162. For a patient with type 2 diabetes, who is mostly sedentary and who has a BMI of 26 and no contraindicative comorbidities, which option below is the best example of a goal that is *realistic* and *attainable*?
   A. "Purchase a pair of walking shoes and walk to and from the mailbox every day."
   B. "Participate in the half marathon at the end of the month"
   C. "Enroll and attend all the daily spin classes at my local health club"
   D. "Walk briskly for 25 minutes every day following dinner"

163. More than 50% of men notice the onset of erectile dysfunction within ten years of the diagnosis of diabetes. Various treatment options are available. Which patient below would *not* be a candidate for phosphodiesterase type 5 inhibitor (PDE5 inhibitor) such as sildenafil (Viagra®), vardenafil (Levitra®), or tadalafil (Cialis®)?
   A. A man with stage 3 chronic kidney disease
   B. A man with moderate liver impairment
   C. A man with mild ischemic heart disease who uses nitroglycerine spray prn for chest pain
   D. All of the above

164. Your patient, a 22 year-old female with type 1 diabetes (diagnosed three years ago), visits with you while home on summer break from college. She reports enjoying college, but realizes that perhaps she has not been as responsible with her diabetes self-care as she really needs to be. Which of the following interventions below is the greatest priority for this patient?
   A. Referral to a nephrologist to check for kidney problems
   B. Referral to an ophthalmologist for an annual dilated eye exam
   C. Referral for MNT for a review of good eating practices, including alcohol consumption
   D. Pre-conception counseling to prevent unplanned pregnancy

165. You are visiting with a patient who has type 1 diabetes and uses an insulin pump. She tells you she is confused about the sick day instructions she has been given and asks why she should increase her basal rate when she so rarely is able to eat anything when she feels sick. Which explanation below is *most* appropriate?
   A. "You are correct to question these instructions. You should never take more insulin when you are not eating, as insulin will drop your blood sugar. Instead of increasing the basal rate, you should actually decrease it. Once you are feeling better and eating normally again, you can resume your regular basal insulin schedule."
   B. "Food is needed to fight the illness and prevent diabetic ketoacidosis (DKA). Extra basal insulin will slowly lower your blood sugar. As your blood sugar drops, you will begin to feel hungry. So in this case, the extra basal insulin actually acts as an appetite stimulant."
   C. "During times of stress such as illness, your liver puts extra glucose into your blood. Your basal insulin covers the glucose from the liver, as opposed to glucose from the carbs you eat. Therefore, extra basal insulin is needed to address the extra liver sugar when you are sick. When you eat or drink something with carbohydrates, you would bolus accordingly."
   D. "We know that because of dehydration, insulin does not get absorbed as well when you are sick. Therefore, in addition to drinking at least 8 oz. of fluid every hour, you must also increase the basal insulin rate to compensate for the decrease in insulin absorption."

166. As of 2013, The American Diabetes Association recommends that bariatric surgery be considered only for those patients with type 2 diabetes who meet which of the following criteria?
   A. Patient has tried numerous dietary and/or behavioral options to lose weight without measureable success
   B. Patient presents with weight-related comorbidities that are potentially life threatening
   C. Patient's BMI ≥ 35 kg/m², and glycemic control through other means has proven difficult
   D. There is no criteria at this time, as the ADA does not recommend bariatric surgery as a treatment option, due to cost and associated risks

167. You receive a referral for a patient, Mr. B., from his primary care provider, for "medication consult and education related to history of non-compliance." Which of the following strategies would provide you with the most accurate and comprehensive assessment on Mr. B's medication knowledge, habits, and associated challenges?
  A. Prepare a written knowledge assessment on which he will match the name of a medication he takes with the appropriate common side effect.
  B. Spend extra time reading through the patient's chart notes by the referring provider to get a better sense of the diabetes medication, education, and adherence history.
  C. Ask the patient to bring a written list of what he is taking and when. Then compare it to the list of what is currently prescribed.
  D. Have the patient bring all the medication he currently takes, in the original container. Then have him describe to you for what purpose, when, and how he takes each medication.

168. Most educators instruct patients to obtain a blood sample from the *side* of the finger when self-monitoring. What is the reason for this advice?
  A. There are more capillaries on the sides of the fingers than the tip, and therefore, easier to get a sufficient sample.
  B. The sides of the fingers have fewer germs, since they do not come in contact with surfaces as much as the tips.
  C. There is less pain when lancing the sides of the fingers, compared to the tips.
  D. Studies have shown that drops obtained from the sides of fingers produce a more accurate whole blood sample result than alternative sites, including fingertips.

169. Which class of oral medications for type 2 diabetes has a mechanism of action that relies on the kidneys to excrete glucose through the urine, and should therefore *not* be used in those with eGFR of less than 30mL/min or by those on dialysis?
  A. Sulfonylureas (i.e. glyburide)
  B. Biguanides (i.e. metformin)
  C. SGLT2 inhibitors (i.e. canagliflozin)
  D. DPP-4 inhibitors (i.e. sitagliptin)

170. Physiologic changes in aging are associated with an increased risk for diabetes and many diabetes-related complications, which may warrant the need for adjustments to the diabetes management plan. Which of the following changes is *not* commonly associated with advanced age?
  A. Reduced metabolic rate that can alter digestion
  B. Increased insulin resistance and decreased insulin effectiveness
  C. Altered pain perception
  D. Decreased renal function

171. Your patient, who uses insulin, is planning to travel. In terms of health and safety, which item below would be the least important for the patient to include in his carry-on luggage?
  A. Snacks, such as nuts and string cheese
  B. Insulin and syringes
  C. Blood glucose meter and extra testing supplies
  D. Diabetic ID and provider contact information

The next four questions refer to the following patient case:

T. M., a 52 year-old Hispanic woman, was diagnosed with type 2 diabetes three weeks ago while hospitalized for dehydration and a bladder infection. She presents for her initial visit with you. Her lab data sent from her PCP show an HbA1c of 8.9%, BMI of 29, and blood pressure controlled with medication. Her PCP has instructed her to take 500 mg metformin twice a day. She states that she has been good about taking her morning dose but forgets about half the time to take her evening dose.

She was given a blood glucose meter in the hospital but is not sure that she is using it correctly. She is not sure when she is supposed to check her blood sugar, so she has been doing it every morning, just before breakfast, when she takes her morning metformin.

Mrs. M seems very sociable and open minded, but admits that she is concerned about this new diagnosis. Her main concern is that she does not want to give up everything she loves to eat, nor have to stop cooking foods her family enjoys. At the advice of her PCP, she is scheduled for a retinal exam next week, but is not sure why because she sees very well, and only needs glasses to see small print.

172. Which of the following DSME topics should be discussed at this visit with Mrs. M.?
   A. Diabetes-related complications and how to prevent them
   B. The meaning of the HbA1c results
   C. How to safely administer insulin
   D. Proper use of an individualized schedule for blood glucose monitoring

173. Based on the information you have so far, which education plan makes the most sense for Mrs. M?
   A. Group classes to include comprehensive diabetes self-management education
   B. One-on-one education sessions, at least until all of her personal concerns are resolved
   C. Printed information on diabetes, including a list of reputable diabetes websites
   D. All of the above are equally appropriate for this patient, provided she has no scheduling conflicts

174. Keeping in mind that Mrs. M has not yet had any diabetes education beyond survival skills, you suggest that she set a preliminary behavioral goal, which the two of you discuss. Based on Mrs. M's current situation, which of the following self-care behavior goals would be appropriate?
   A. Lose 10 pounds by the next visit (3 months from now)
   B. Take metformin as directed, with fewer missed doses, over the next three months
   C. Reduce HbA1c to less than 8% by the next three-month visit
   D. Significantly reduce the risk of diabetes-related complications

175. What referrals, if any, should be made at this time for Mrs. M.?
   A. Mental health (to address her anxieties)
   B. Ophthalmology (since she has just been diagnosed with type 2 diabetes)
   C. Registered dietitian to address her meal concerns and weight management
   D. No referrals are warranted until she has at least completed initial DSME

176. What are the ADA-recommended cholesterol goals (2013) for adults with diabetes and no history of cardiovascular disease?
    A. LDL < 100 mg/dL, HDL > 40 mg/dL (men) and > 50 mg/dL (women), triglycerides < 150 mg/dL
    B. LDL < 150 mg/dL, HDL > 40 mg/dL (men) and > 50 mg/dL (women), triglycerides < 180 mg/dL
    C. Total cholesterol < 200, HDL > 40 mg/dL, triglycerides < 100 mg/dL
    D. LDL < 150 mg/dL, HDL > 50 mg/dL (men) and > 40 mg/dL (women), triglycerides < 100 mg/dL

177. According to recently revised Medicare guidelines, a referral for medical nutrition therapy (MNT) by a registered dietitian can be made by whom?
    A. Any credentialed or certified member of the diabetes care team, including the certified diabetes educator
    B. A member of the diabetes care team with any of the following credentials: physician, qualified non-physician practitioner (NP/PA), or pharmacist
    C. Only a primary care provider, including the treating physician or qualified non-physician practitioner (NP or PA)
    D. Only the treating physician

178. Which of the following options below is a *modifiable* risk factor for type 2 diabetes?
    A. Weight/obesity
    B. Family history
    C. Race/ethnicity
    D. Age

179. You are conducting a seminar for family members and significant others of those with diabetes. In your advice for this group, what would you describe as the primary question a support person should ask him/herself?
    A. "What will help this person with diabetes gain greater control of his/her chronic disease?"
    B. "What can I do that will result in better blood sugars for this person with diabetes?"
    C. "What does this person with diabetes want in the way of support?"
    D. "What can I do or say that will result in a longer, complication-free life for this person with diabetes?"

180. Identify the statement below that is *true* with regards to recommended lab values.
    A. Someone with an HDL of 31 mg/dL is not at risk for CVD as long as the total cholesterol is not above 200 mg/dL.
    B. A serum creatinine of 3.6 mg/dL in a 55-year-old female indicates probable renal impairment.
    C. Regardless of regular SMBG values, someone with type 1 diabetes with an HbA1c of 5.9% is well controlled.
    D. A patient who has a creatinine level of less than 56 IU/L does not have fatty liver disease.

181. Which of the following personal characteristics has proven to positively affect behavioral outcomes through healthy coping to one's diabetes?
    A. Stubbornness
    B. Affluence
    C. Optimism
    D. Consistency

182. What is the main difference between *process evaluation* (or *process*) and *summative* (or *outcomes*) *evaluation*?
  A. Process evaluation deals with patients and summative evaluation deals with the organization.
  B. The purpose of process evaluation is to make needed adjustments to the educational process; the purpose of summative evaluation is to determine the effectiveness of the education process.
  C. The scope of formative evaluation is small, as in a single session or class, whereas the summative evaluation encompasses a period of time (usually one year) and includes statistics on an organization's productivity (i.e. number of patients served, classes taught, etc.).
  D. The object of formative evaluation is to identify gaps or deficits and then make changes and adjustments as needed; the object of summative evaluation is to compile and summarize data for reporting purposes.

183. In response to low patient satisfaction scores for the class on medications, the diabetes educator redesigns the class content outline to contain more information on the mechanism of action of each class of oral medication. After receiving approval from the continuous quality improvement (CQI) team, the educator implements the new content. She is surprised when the patient satisfaction scores for the class are even lower the next month. What is the most likely explanation for the failure of this change to better satisfy participants?
  A. The educator most likely failed to thoroughly explain her idea to the CQI team.
  B. The educator did not collect and analyze information on why the patients did not like the class before deciding on the change.
  C. The evaluation method used to gauge patient satisfaction is most likely not a valid or reliable tool.
  D. The educator was not creative in her solution to the problem.

184. Mr. D drops by the clinic on his way home from work to obtain a copy of his wife's most recent lab results. You know that Mr. D comes to appointments with his wife and assists in her diabetes self-management. What is the appropriate action for you to take?
  A. Politely explain that it is a HIPAA violation to provide any private health information to anyone but the individual or personal representative (someone legally appointed to make healthcare decisions)
  B. Provide Mr. D with a blank copy of the Release of Information form and tell him that if his wife will sign it, only then will you be able to comply with his request
  C. Suggest that the lab is not needed at this time and that it can be discussed with the provider or educator in person at Mrs. D's next appointment
  D. Since Mrs. D has identified her husband as a participant in her care, you may provide Mr. D with a copy of the lab result, provided it does not violate the policies of your workplace

185. The American Association of Diabetes Educators' Policy and Advocacy group has identified six goals. Which of the following choices is *not* one of the identified goals?
  A. Influencing the future of diabetes education and the role of the diabetes educator in health care
  B. Limiting the specialized skill of providing evidence-based diabetes education to health care professionals who are certified as diabetes educators
  C. Advocating for policies that improve access to diabetes self-management training
  D. Attaining and maintaining reasonable reimbursement for diabetes educators

186. Which of the following examples violates infection control principles?
  A. A patient uses soap and water instead of alcohol to clean the skin before administering an insulin injection
  B. A clinic uses one blood glucose meter to perform all point of care glucose tests for patients
  C. An inpatient diabetes educator trains all patients on pen use with a single demo pen, but changes the pen needle each time
  D. Parents who have two children with type 1 diabetes withdraw insulin from the same insulin vial but with a separate and new sterile insulin syringe for each child's dose

187. What is the distinction between *assessment* and *evaluation*?
  A. Assessment is clinical in nature, whereas evaluation is typically administrative.
  B. Assessment is always done at the beginning of a process or procedure, whereas evaluation is performed at the end.
  C. Assessment implies gathering and interpreting data for the purpose of directing action, whereas evaluation is to determine the extent to which an action or process was successful.
  D. In relation to diabetes program management, there is no significant difference between assessment and evaluation; the two are used interchangeably.

188. Which of the following marketing strategies has been found to be the most reliable and cost-effective method of bringing new patients into a diabetes education program?
  A. Radio ads
  B. Personal outreach to referring providers
  C. Word of mouth (current participants, employees, etc.)
  D. Finding and contacting patients who were previously hospitalized and experienced hyperglycemia

189. National Diabetes Awareness month presents an annual opportunity to promote diabetes advocacy through community outreach activities. What month is National Diabetes Awareness month?
  A. January
  B. April
  C. September
  D. November

190. Which of the following options below is the *most* appropriate example of a learning objective for your class?
  A. Learner will select an appropriate, balanced meal choice from a restaurant menu
  B. Learner will know what it means to eat healthily
  C. Learner will improve HbA1c through better food choices
  D. Learner will understand the difference between glycemic index and glycemic load

191. You are preparing to teach an introductory course at a community center on nutrition intervention as part of diabetes care. Which of the following materials would be *most* appropriate for the class you will be teaching?
   A. Copies of ADA guidelines on nutrition
   B. Models of foods, nutrition labels, and sample restaurant menus
   C. Graphs showing rates of diabetes complication for different HbA1c levels
   D. Props to demonstrate personal foot care (mirror, file, socks, types of shoes, etc.)

192. You have been asked to teach a diabetes class to a small group of patients, all of whom are hearing impaired. You have secured an American Sign Language (ASL) translator to interpret for the class members. What other modification should be made to meet the needs of this particular audience?
   A. Write medication names and other "proper" nouns on the white board.
   B. Modify some of the handouts to include more pictures and less text.
   C. Arrange all chairs in a circle so class members can clearly see each other.
   D. Provide each class member with a pad of paper and pen to facilitate written communication.

The next two questions pertain to the following scenario:

> A diabetes educator works at several different diabetes care centers, spread throughout the state. In preparation for individualizing her interventions for the needs of each center's population, she is conducting population needs assessment for each of the centers.

193. Which geographic areas are most underserved in terms of access to diabetes education?
   A. Inner cities
   B. Suburban areas
   C. Rural areas, particularly in the South
   D. States with the highest population density

194. Which of the following statements relating to barriers to diabetes education is *true*?
   A. Most primary care providers do not agree that their patients need more education and support for diabetes.
   B. Patients over the age of 65 are more likely to seek diabetes education than their middle-aged counter parts.
   C. Reflecting the makeup of the diabetes population, the majority of participants in DSME programs are minorities.
   D. Tension and disagreement between primary care providers and diabetes educators regarding self-care recommendations has been found to be a barrier to patients' access to diabetes education.

195. You discover that the middle school your patient attends does not permit him to carry his blood glucose meter or insulin with him. What step below would you take to advocate for your patient?
   A. Teach the patient how he should check his glucose so as to stay within the school guidelines (i.e. before and after school)
   B. Show the patient ways he can hide his testing and insulin supplies and perform the necessary skills in the bathroom, so as not to get in trouble
   C. Contact the school principal, school nurse, and head district nurse to get clarification on the policy and explain the need for modification for your patient
   D. Encourage the mother of the patient to contact the school board or her legislator if necessary

196. "The systematic process by which the worth or value of something, in the case of DSME teaching or learning is judged" is known as which of the following?
   A. Evaluation
   B. Documentation
   C. Planning
   D. Implementation

197. Standard 10 of National Standards for Diabetes Self-management and Support (2013) states that DSME providers "will measure the effectiveness of the education and support and look for ways to improve any identified gaps in services or service quality." As a *first* step in the continuous quality improvement process, the educator should ask which one of the following questions?
   A. Are the methods used to provide patients with the services they need and want effective?
   B. What programs or initiatives should be implemented to improve outcomes?
   C. How will we measure the effectiveness of a change or initiative?
   D. What resources will be needed to implement changes to current practice?

198. Which of the following entities is *not* an organization that accredits or officially "recognizes" diabetes self-management education programs – a necessary requirement for Medicare reimbursement?
   A. The National Certification Board for Diabetes Educators (NCBDE)
   B. The American Diabetes Association (ADA)
   C. The American Association of Diabetes Educators (AADE)
   D. All of the above are organizations that can recognize or accredit DSME programs

199. Which of the following aggregate patient outcomes are required to be collected and reported as part of DSME program recognition and accreditation?
   A. Patient attendance rates for educational appointments
   B. Overall change in patient HbA1c (pre/post education)
   C. Percent of patients achieving behavioral goals
   D. The AADE and ADA do not specify which outcomes must be tracked

200 .In 2007 researchers observed community-based diabetes screenings at 12 separate health fairs in Harlem, New York City. The results, published in 2010, revealed several concerns, which may apply to community-based diabetes screening fairs throughout the country. Which of the following statements was *not* a finding of this research (and likely not a common concern related to local diabetes health fairs)?

A. Due to a general lack of trust in of health care professionals, attendance at local health fairs is usually poor and therefore a deterrent to holding such events.

B. Screeners typically use equipment that is designed for home use only, and is not intended for diagnostic or screening purposes.

C. Technique of screeners tends to vary, which can skew test results.

D. Screening rarely includes gathering diabetes risk assessment data or recent caloric intake (fasting status).

Answers and Explanations

1. **A: Assessment.** The other steps in the DSME process (in order) are: goal setting, planning, implementation, and evaluation/monitoring. Diagnosis and referral, while necessary, are not considered official steps in the diabetes self-management education process.

2. **C:** Keeping a physical activity log was associated with a higher level of self efficacy in a small-scale 2006 study. Those in the record-keeping group did not have significantly higher levels of physical activity than those who did not keep a record over the six-week intervention period. They did, however, report feeling positive about record-keeping, stating that it helped them to think more about personal activity and it was not overly time consuming. There is no evidence that activity record keeping is associated with increased regimen adherence, gym memberships or class enrollment, or perceived barriers to physical activity.

3. **A:** A stress test with ECG may be warranted, as this person is over 40, previously sedentary, has risk factors for CVD, and is beginning a program that is more intense than brisk walking, which is mild in intensity. The DEXA scan and the ankle-brachial index are not necessary based on the information given.

4. **B:** Demonstrating a skill such as insulin administration allows the patient to learn by watching, listening, and then doing. The return demonstration also allows the educator to witness the patient's level of competency and then correct mistakes. This teaching strategy takes a bit more time, and works best in one-on-one situations or in small groups, but is the most effective way to both teach and assess a clinical skill. A written quiz may be a way to assess knowledge but does not enable the educator to assess the patient's technique, nor does it provide the best opportunity to instruct. A video or printed handout can instruct to a certain extent, but neither provides a means of assessing the patient's ability to self-administer insulin. These tools are best used to reinforce the demonstration. While verbal acknowledgement of understanding may be part of the assessment, it is not sufficient to assess a patient's level of understanding and competency of a self-care skill such as insulin administration.

5. **C:** Cultural characteristics/barriers of your population are addressed in many ways, among them: asking about food preferences and restrictions, inviting family participation, and moderating your speech rate and tone. Keep in mind that what may be culturally sensitive to one culture could be offensive to another. This underscores the importance of knowing your patient population. While readiness for change, low literacy/numeracy, and poor support are important considerations, they are not addressed by the policies described in the scenario.

6. **B:** According to the 2008 consensus statement on managing pregnancy with pre-existing diabetes, optimal glucose targets are: pre-meal/fasting glucose: 60 to 99 mg/dL; peak postprandial: <129 mg/dL; HbA1c <6%. Option (A) is too stringent, and options (C) and (D) are not stringent enough. Note that for pregnancy, glucose is not considered hypoglycemia until the level is less than 60 mg/dL, although this may need to be adjusted for each individual.

7. **A:** Providing materials and experiences to enhance her knowledge and skills will best address this patient's lack of confidence of success. While addressing psychosocial needs is important, these responses do not correlate with this action. Highlighting the benefits of good diabetes management is incorrect because this action would be more appropriate if the patient rated the importance to make a change as low. The patient is already convinced of the importance, and highlighting benefits is not the priority. Finally, it is not unusual for patients to believe it is very important to change but

to have low confidence in the ability to do so. This may be due to a lack of knowledge, skill or self-confidence.

8. D: Misplacement of small items, such as glucose meters was not one of the barriers reposted by patients in a recent survey (Tenderich, 2013). Common barriers do include cost, discomfort, lack of proper instruction and ongoing support, as well as others: physical limitation (dexterity/visual disability), cognitive deficits, time constraints and inconvenience, and emotional components such as stress or anxiety.

9. D: The medication regimen is the most important factor to consider when assessing risk for hypoglycemia in relation to exercise. Insulin and insulin secretagogues are the greatest risk factor; in the absence any of these medications, risk for hypoglycemia with exercise is low. For patients who use these medications, food intake may be adjusted and careful consideration should be given to preventing, predicting, recognizing, and treating hypoglycemia.

10. D: The patient denies that she has diabetes and disagrees with the doctor's referral for DSME. This is a sign that she is resistant to accept her diagnosis and that she is not ready to make changes in light of it. A tearful patient may be feeling overwhelmed or sad because she believes she will have to give up favorite foods. It may also be that she is not ready to change, but not necessarily. Option (B) is incorrect because, while not speaking may at times indicate an unwillingness to change, the patient may also be concentrating on the demonstration. Option (C), incorrectly answering review questions, may be an indication that the patient misunderstood or did not see or hear the material, but is not necessarily unwilling to change. The fact that she responded indicates that she is at least engaged.

11. A: It is *not* true that medical nutrition therapy is recommended for only those persons with diabetes who are underweight, overweight, or obese. In fact, MNT is recommended for anyone who has diabetes, regardless of nutritional status. In addition, a registered dietitian should be closely involved with a patient's diabetes care plan to assist with individualized meal planning in many cases, such as: if the patient is a child with celiac disease, hospitalized, or pregnant; if the patient has co-morbidities affected by diet, or if the patient has prediabetes.

12. C: Milking the lanced finger at the tip can obstruct blood flow. In addition, it may skew the results by increasing the amount of interstitial fluid in the sample. A patient should milk the finger closer to the base of the finger and move towards the tip, or milk the finger before lancing. All other choices are acceptable actions. Soap and water is preferred over alcohol, as alcohol is unnecessary and may actually skew the sample. Puncture depth may be set to the patient's preference as long as a sufficient drop is produced. The shallower the depth setting, the less pain there will be. Patients should be encouraged to use a system of recording results that fits them best.

13. D: Hypertension is the condition that will suffer the most from the patient's meal due to the high sodium content. Choice (A), hyperlipidemia, is addressed due to the low amount of saturated fat. Choice (B), type 2 diabetes, is addressed due to the moderate amount of carbohydrates (about 50 grams). Choice (C), obesity, is also addressed by the reasonable amount of total calories in the meal.

14. C: The bargaining stage is characterized by inaccurate explanations and/or erroneous cures. The patient "makes a deal" with self, provider, God, or others to get rid of the diabetes. Extremes of compulsive behavior often accompany this stage. Denial is characterized by disbelief in the diagnosis; anger is characterized by irritation, rage, anxicty, or guilt. Frustration and depression can occur at any time and are characterized by feelings of hopelessness and trouble establishing or

maintaining good self-care habits. Acceptance is the stage at which the patient becomes involved in his or her care and requests information and help to improve.

15. D: Small group discussion around a table where patients teach each other a skill after seeing it demonstrated by the educator is an instruction strategy that addresses visual, auditory, and tactile learning styles. The interaction (teaching back) makes it memorable; studies show that people remember best when they not only see and hear something, but also when they say and do it. All other options are good strategies, but are not likely to lead to the best retention.

16. B: Limited literacy skills are the strongest predictors of health status – stronger than ethnicity, income level, age, and other factors.

17. B: The calorie balance/surplus (total calorie intake vs. calorie expenditure) has proven to be the most important aspect of weight loss. Other important elements include adherence to diet and enthusiasm of the counselor. Composition of nutrients, glycemic index, and fiber have not been shown to affect weight loss as much as energy deficit.

18. B: Level of family support, while very important to assess, is not considered an element of patient knowledge. Choices (A) literacy/numeracy, (B) previous DSME, and (D) proficiency of self-care skills are all important elements to assess in order to gauge the patient's knowledge and ability to gain knowledge.

19. D: All of the above should be noted. A medication regimen should include all prescription, over-the-counter medications, vitamins, and complementary and alternative therapies.

20. A: The breakfast meal is definitely the most unbalanced. The meal consists of almost all carbohydrates and total carbohydrates are over 120 grams (twice the normally recommended amount for most men). While lunch and dinner may be on the large side in terms of serving sizes and total calories, they are at least balanced between protein, fat, and carbs, and both have closer to the typically recommended amount of carbohydrates.

21. B: Rephrase to "How do you hope that learning more about diabetes will help you?" The patient may need clarification on what you mean by diabetes education-related goals. Choice (A) is belittling and will put the patient on the defensive. Choice (C) is incorrect because he is awaiting information from you. While silence is appropriate while a patient thinks, it is not appropriate when he has expressed that he needs more information. Choice (D) is not the best choice because you are suggesting options ("putting words in his mouth"), rather than allowing the patient to state what really matters to him.

22. B: A visual learner is most likely to prefer and/or benefit from seeing, watching, or reading, to include visual demonstrations and visual aids as well as reinforcement through reading materials. Choices (C) and (D) represent auditory/verbal instructional methods. While role-playing is partially verbal and partially auditory (and partially tactile), it is more action oriented and may therefore be distracting to a strictly visual learner.

23. A: A BMI of anything less than 18.5 is underweight. A BMI of 18.5 to 24.9 is normal weight. A BMI of 25 to 29.9 is overweight. A BMI of 30 and above is obese, with over 40 being extremely or morbidly obese.

24. B: Food records provide the data by which the current nutrition plan and adherence to that plan may be evaluated by both the patient keeping the record and the educator/provider who reviews it with the patient. While a personal review of the record may encourage the patient, it is not the main purpose. Insurance providers do not require a personal food log, as the RD notes are sufficient documentation. While record keeping is important in diabetes, development of this habit is not the main purpose of keeping a food log, nor is forcing the person to pay more attention to what he/she eats, although that is certainly an added benefit.

25. C: The situation that describes driving while experiencing hypoglycemia symptoms is the best choice to assess a patient's ability to deal with a glucose emergency. Hypothetical situations are excellent ways to assess a patient's diabetes knowledge; however, you must construct situations that will test the type of knowledge you are trying to assess. Choice (A) would assess a patient's ability to make appropriate food choices. Choice (B) deals with problem solving related to travel and how to acquire medication, and choice (D) addresses the healthy coping skill of dealing with friends who mean well but are misinformed.

26. D: The patient should prime the needle before dialing the dose for each and every injection. This is to expel any air in the pen and to "prime" the pen tip with insulin. There is no need to clean the skin with alcohol, as long as the skin is clean. Likewise, pinching of the skin is not necessary unless the patient is very thin or a child. Even then, with the smaller length of pen needle, pinching is not usually needed. After injecting insulin, the patient should leave the needle in the skin for about ten seconds to ensure all the insulin has been delivered. This is a step that many patients forget or were never taught because it is a variation on administration with a syringe.

27. B: An interpersonal barrier may include struggles with family, peers, or with healthcare team members. In this case, that patient's interpersonal struggles relate to her ability to eat healthfully. Other types of barriers include personal (co-morbidities, physical disability, poor coping skills, and inaccurate health beliefs) and environmental (financial constraints, job-related issues, transportation issues, safety of environment, other priorities). These other types are represented in choices A, C, and D, but are not the best choices for the scenario described because they do not focus on relationship with the patient's family members.

28. A: The Social Cognitive Theory maintains that individuals learn from their personal experiences as well as from observing the actions and experiences of others. SCT addresses psychosocial factors that influence health behavior and methods of stimulating behavioral change. The Health Belief Model stipulates that a person's decision to change health behavior depends on several factors, including level of personal vulnerability, belief in seriousness of the problem, belief in effectiveness of the change, associated costs of the change, presence of action cues, and level of self efficacy. The Theory of Planned Behavior applies three major constructs: attitudes towards the desired behavior, perceived societal view of the behavior, and the knowledge/skill level of the person. The Transtheoretical Model (TTM) states that change is likely to occur only when the patient has reached a stage at which he or she is ready to change. The stages of the TTM are: precontemplation, contemplation, preparation, action, maintenance, and termination.

29. B: Lack of interest on the part of patients was not identified as a major barrier to optimal care for patients with diabetes. The other choices listed: low health literacy, limited time to see the provider, and complexity of diabetes education were all identified themes. Other themes included difficulty navigating the healthcare system, diagnosis not leading directly to DSME, episodic versus comprehensive focus, and patient education being undervalued by the healthcare system and payers.

30. D: Seeing a nephrologist annually in the absence of hypertension or kidney problems is not necessary. The primary care provider or endocrinologist can check blood pressure and kidney function and then refer if a problem is identified. According to ADA Standards of Medical Care – 2013, regular dental visits, an annual dilated eye exam to check for retinopathy, and annual lipid screening tests are all part of recommended components of comprehensive diabetes care.

31. C: Smoking status, along with readiness to quit should be assessed at every visit.

32. C: Diminished or absent pedal pulses indicate poor circulation. All other choices are normal findings for a lower extremity assessment. Note that pulse palpation often has false positives and false negatives, so one must practice the technique in order to prevent erroneous assessment findings.

33. C: Flexibility exercise, or stretching, should be considered in the fitness plan, as it can provide fitness benefits such as increasing joint range of motion and stability for older adults. However, flexibility exercise should not take the place of aerobic and resistance exercise. It has been questioned whether or not flexibility training may decrease injury, but this has not been proven. The other types of exercise include aerobic exercise for cardiovascular health and resistance exercises for muscle strength and core conditioning, which improve glycemic control and increase mobility. Both are being addressed in the patient's current plan. Toning exercise is not an official exercise category.

34. A: The patient who records all information in her spiral notebook is the best example of good SMBG record keeping, regardless of the condition of her book. The information she has recorded will enable her (as well as the healthcare team members) to get a complete picture of how her glucose responds to food, activity, medication doses, etc. By recording dates and times, she will be able to identify patterns more easily, as will the educator/provider. The other answer choices are each missing an important component: by not keeping a written record, the patient is missing the important factors (food, activity, medicine) that may help explain and ultimately improve the readings. The patient who does not bring her meter to her appointment is missing the opportunity to have the meter tested for accuracy, and does not allow the healthcare team the opportunity to download it (to confirm her recordings are accurate and complete and view helpful summary report data), or to assess her SMBG technique. A patient record that does not indicate the days on which the readings were taken is at a great disadvantage because both the patient and the educator will be unable to associate the readings with what was happening at the time, including food and medication (since he did not record those items with his readings).

35. B: Inviting the client's wife to help recall what he ate yesterday would be appropriate in this case. Family members can often be helpful when gathering information for the assessment. If you were testing his diabetes knowledge and the patient was unable to answer a question, then "pt. does not answer" should be noted. (A) would be appropriate, but you are seeking to find out what the client actually ate. A 24-hour dietary recall is an appropriate tool in some cases, but your initial assessment is more of an overview, and the information can be provided by means less burdensome to the patient. Finally, choice (D) would not ever be appropriate because of the use of a patronizing title and question.

36. D: A serum creatinine of 2.8 mg/dL should raise a red flag, as it indicates likely renal impairment. Although estimated glomerular filtration rate (eGFR) is calculated with additional factors such as age, sex, race, and weight, the creatinine of this patient is not in the normal range for

any demographic. The FDA recommends against using metformin for any serum creatinine above 1.5 mg/dL due to a likelihood of renal impairment. Estimated GFR calculators are available online and typically use the MDRD Study Equation or the Cockroft-Gault Equation. Refer this patient to nephrology immediately. Although the A1c and LDL levels are considered slightly above ideal for most patients, they are not to the level of immediate concern. The HDL of 88 is high, but for HDL the goal is to have a high value: above 40 for men and above 50 for women. Therefore, the HDL is not a concern.

37. C: Relying on the color of a medication, along with saying "I forgot my glasses," or using pictures drawn on the bottles, etc. are all signs of possible health literacy barriers. Financial barriers could be indicated by a patient skipping doses or cutting doses in half, or by delaying picking up prescriptions. Cognitive barriers would be indicated by a patient exhibiting confusion or forgetfulness; fear of side effects might be the cause of a patient who does not take medication at all, or continues to take a lesser dose than recommended. If any barrier or adherence issue is suspected, the educator should investigate further by using open-ended, non-judgmental questions.

38. A: Acanthosis nigricans is a darkening and thickening of the skin, typically on the back/sides of the neck or the axillae; indicative of insulin resistance. Option (B) describes Kussmaul breathing. Darkening of the toenails is not a recognized condition, except in *subungual hematoma (which occurs when a nail is traumatized and blood forms under the nail).* Option (D) is eschar. (

39. A: Talking to the nurse of the referring provider and using the information to complete the assessment form is the *least* effective and least recommended way to complete the initial assessment. While gathering information from referring providers may be helpful, the bulk of the information assessment should come from the patient or your direct observation of the patient. All other answer choices: face-to-face meeting (with family members), completion of an electronic form prior to visit, and group assessment with individuals completing personal information on their own are all acceptable methods to conduct initial DSME assessments.

40. A: Glyburide is a sulfonylurea, an insulin secretagogue with a comparatively high rate of hypoglycemia. This medication should not be taken if the person does not intend to eat that day. In addition, basal insulin is usually taken in a full or reduced amount, even when the person is NPO, as it is basal and basal insulin addresses primarily hepatic glucose. Other answer choices all indicate correct understanding. Lantus® (glargine) can be kept at room temperature for the duration of its use. Metformin does not require food, as it will not cause a drop in glucose lower than a normal level. Insulin in a vial or pen should not be used beyond the recommended amount of time, which for NovoLog (as well as most insulins) is 28 days.

41. A: "My mother believes I got diabetes from eating too much candy as a kid" is not part of the health history, but rather may speak to the family dynamics and support. All other choices would be more important to note, including choice (D), which gives the duration of diabetes.

42. D: Sexual orientation is not information collected during the initial assessment, as stipulated in National Standards for DSME. Although level of family support is assessed, this does not extend to the nature of sexual orientation. The other choices: financial status, emotional response, and cultural influences are all part of the information gathered, along with many other factors.

43. B: A patient with a BMI of 41 kg/m² is morbidly obese. Any BMI over 40 is categorized as morbid obesity, with BMI over 49 as super obesity. Morbid obesity is now defined according to the BMI. Choice (A) may not meet the criteria for morbid obesity as we do not have the patient's height

and cannot therefore calculate a BMI. Typically, someone with morbid obesity is at least 100 pounds overweight. Choice (C) says nothing about the patient's weight or BMI. The fact that the patient is considering bariatric surgery does not automatically indicate morbid obesity. The patient in choice (D) is not the correct option as there is only information about weight; his BMI could be normal if he is 6'9", overweight if he is 6'3", obese if he is 5'8", or morbidly obese if he is 5'3". Without the height information, the patient described in choice (D) cannot be classified.

44. D: Presenting a scenario that is applicable to the patient will give the clinician an opportunity to observe whether or not the patient has the capability to make the calculations necessary for safe and appropriate action. The patient's grade level and his math grades are not indicative of current skill or ability level. Asking the patient to self-report numeracy problems is unreliable because the patient may give an inaccurate self-assessment due to embarrassment or he may not realize that he even struggles with numeracy. Assigning a take-home math test runs the risk that the patient will have someone else complete it or help with completing, and it is likely to miss specific areas/topics that currently apply to this specific patient.

45. C: Annual influenza vaccination and hepatitis B vaccination for adults less than 60 yrs is an ADA-recommended Standard of Care in Diabetes (2013). For those unvaccinated adults who are 60 years or older, the hepatitis B vaccination should be considered, but evidence of cost effectiveness is still lacking for older adults. Other choices are only partially correct. An echocardiogram is not recommended annually as a Standard of Care. A dilated eye exam is recommended at diagnosis for those with type 2 diabetes and within 5 years of onset for those with type 1 diabetes. Repeat exams should be performed annually (more often if needed), rather than every six months. The C-peptide exam is sometimes used to differentiate type 2 from type 1 diabetes, to assess endogenous insulin production, or to qualify a patient for insulin pump therapy (insurance provider requirement), but is not recommended as a Standard of Care.

46. A: Medicare guidelines do not justify individual sessions for diabetes education simply because the patient prefers one-on-one education. There must be a documented rationale, such as unavailability of classes, physical or cultural barriers, or another physician-documented need to provide reimbursement for one-on-one classes.

47. D: A financial barrier is the most probable obstacle facing this patient, based on the limited information available. The patient takes her medication consistently, but cuts the expensive name-brand pill in half. She was willing to add more vegetables, but not the more pricey fresh vegetables. Of course, the clinician should never assume a barrier without having an honest, frank discussion with the patient first. A transportation barrier might be the case since she only uses canned vegetables (perhaps not to travel to the store as often), but this does not explain why she cuts only one of her medicines in half. There is no evidence of a cultural or cognitive barrier in the information provided, although again, these should not be ruled out without talking to the patient first.

48. C: Acknowledge his reluctance and ask if he might be willing to share some of his knowledge and experiences with the other class members. By acknowledging his emotional state, you validate his feelings, which will help him feel that you are not his opponent. By asking him to share his knowledge, you invite him to participate in a way that does not contradict his perception but will still allow him to experience the class. Option (A) is sometimes appropriate if the patient insists he will not attend (if option C fails), but the patient should not be dismissed so easily. Option (B) puts the person on the defensive, and may possibly embarrass him. This will damage rapport between the patient and the clinician and he will be less likely to want to attend. Option (D) is

avoiding/deflecting the clinician's responsibility and puts the spouse in the middle of the educator patient-relationship.

49. B: Testing only when the numbers look good misses the point of self-monitoring. The purpose of self-monitoring is to provide the patient with "immediate feedback and data, enabling persons with diabetes to make changes in their management plans and reinforcing of challenging current lifestyle behaviors" (ref. 1, p. 168). By only monitoring at times when the numbers look good, the patient misses the opportunity to make corrections at times that will ultimately improve overall glycemic control. On the other hand, it is appropriate for patients to monitor when they do not feel well, overnight when they are concerned about a change to basal insulin, and two hours post prandial.

50. C: Reporting progress is not a critical educator skill when assessing a patient's ability to plan goals. Monitoring progress is an important part of the goals process, but not in assessing one's ability to *plan*. The four critical skills for assessing patients' planning skills are: interpret information gathering, facilitating engagement, hypothesis testing, and problem analysis.

51. C: Preparation is the stage represented by this patient's words and actions. He has not yet actively engaged in the behavior change he needs – the action stage, but is no longer unaware of the problem – the precontemplation stage. He has even moved beyond just acknowledging there is a problem that he may want to do something about – the contemplation stage, to actually making plans that will facilitate behavior change – the preparation stage.

52. A: Nausea and subsequent weight loss are not chief fears of patients who are being prescribed insulin, as they are not common side effects. It is however, a common side effect for some GLP-1 agonist injectable medications. Other common concerns include the idea that taking insulin will actually make diabetes worse or lead to complications (even though the opposite is true), fear of needles, and fear of hypoglycemia. Other commonly reported concerns include social stigma and possible weight gain.

53. A: Visual and tactile/dexterity issues are a possible concern for this patient. She squints and is not attempting to complete the written paperwork, which may indicate that she cannot see well. Her shaking hands indicate that small movements, such as those needed to check blood sugar, administer insulin, or even hold a pen, could be tricky. Option (B) is not the best choice because based on your observation, you have no reason to suspect a hearing impairment. Likewise, she has not given indications thus far of a financial barrier or a cultural barrier. While you should not rule out the possibilities of other learning barriers, option (A) is the best choice because you have already seen indications that these may be present.

54. B: This response is an accurate description of the difference between type 1 and type 2 diabetes, specifically, why oral medications work on the latter but not the former. The other options are partially true, but also include fallacies. Option (A) claims that insulin is used for type 1 diabetes primarily for weight gain. This is false. Option (C) states that type 1 is more severe than type 2. This is a fallacy. Severity is a measure of level of control, not type. Option (D) suggests that oral medications would be effective (if too drastic) for lowering blood glucose of someone with type 1. This is not true. Oral medication would have little or no effect and would not sustain the person with type 1 diabetes.

55. C: It is not necessary for a person with diabetes to eat every time he or she drives. However, if the person is at risk for a hypoglycemia reaction, such as by recently exercising or if his or her

insulin is scheduled to peak, then this may become an important action. Patients should always check their glucose before operating a vehicle; they should never operate a vehicle if a reading is close to hypoglycemic. Other safety precautions include wearing medical identification, stopping every one to two hours to monitor, and carrying testing supplies and a source of glucose.

56. D: Demonstration is an active-learning instructional strategy in which the educator has a good amount of control over content because he or she first performs the demonstration. Options (A) and (B) are active-learning instructional strategies that enhance learning, but over which the educator has less control of content. These are participant driven to a greater extent than demonstration. Option (C) is a passive-learning instructional strategy. Although this strategy affords the educator a great deal of control over content, it does not involve the learner to a great extent and therefore, typically yields less retention and understanding than more active-learning instructional strategies.

57. A: Activity-related hypoglycemia may occur up to 24 hours after an intense activity is stopped. With intense or prolonged activity, the glycogen stores are depleted. In these situations, the patient may need to consume a moderate amount of carbohydrates during and/or within two hours after the activity to restore muscle glycogen. While all other choices are certainly within the window of concern, they do not cover the whole time span at which exercise-related hypoglycemia can occur.

58. D: Thiazolidinediones (TZD) medications, such as pioglitazone (Actos®) can take 12 to 16 weeks to reach maximum effect; many patients may notice no difference after only one month. At this point, neither a different medication nor a higher dose is warranted. It is possible that the patient may have gained weight with the medication, as it is a reported side effect. This does not necessarily mean that the patient is eating more, as often the weight gain is due to increased water retention. The educator should assess for edema in the lower extremities and consult with the provider on an appropriate diuretic or dose alteration if edema is present.

59. B: This response is the best example of *developing discrepancy* in motivational interviewing. The idea is that the inconsistency between a behavior/belief and the desired outcome will spur the patient to conclude that it is worth the struggle to make changes. In this case, the educator acknowledges the struggle and the discrepancy between the two sides of the argument and then helps the patient focus on the long-term outcome of fewer complications and better health. Option (A) does not validate the patient's struggles, but rather dismisses them. In addition, it does not highlight the positive outcome that may result if the patient does monitor. Option (C) somewhat acknowledges the struggle by pointing out that many experience the same thing, but the response does not highlight discrepancy. Option (D) praises the patient, which is important, but skips over the patient's comments entirely. It does not acknowledge the struggle or point out the discrepancy between the current thought and desired outcome.

60. B: When a patient has changed behavior to adopt self-care strategies, he or she could relapse into old habits. The diabetes educator can assist in the prevention, recognition, and addressing of behavioral relapse. Teaching the patient to be self-aware and to have a plan to deal with stressful situations is an appropriate educator strategy to prevent relapse. The American Diabetes Association (2013) recommends intervention by a health professional when a patient exhibits signs of "gross disregard for the medical regimen, depression, possibility of self-harm, debilitating anxiety, indications of an eating disorder, or cognitive functioning that significantly impairs judgment."

61. C: Patients with unstable proliferative retinopathy should not include strength training, weight lifting, or high-impact activities in the exercise regimen because the resulting excessive systolic blood pressure response may further damage vessels in the eyes. Patients with proliferative retinopathy will have significant restrictions to exercise, although some physical activity is still recommended, beyond just activities of daily living. Swimming, walking, low-impact dancing, and stationary cycling are some examples of recommended activities. While a stress test is recommended before beginning an exercise program for those of high risk, this test mainly assesses risks related to coronary artery disease, peripheral vascular disease, and autonomic neuropathy. Passing a stress test would not necessarily indicate safety of exercise for someone with proliferative retinopathy.

62. D: Sulfonamide medications compete with sulfonylurea medications, such as glipizide, for protein binding sites, thereby keeping more of the glipizide acting in the blood stream. This can result in hypoglycemia. Corticosteroid medications tend to raise blood sugars, especially post-prandial blood sugars. This effect is more on the intrinsic disease than on other medications. Likewise, protease inhibitors (antiviral drugs) such as indinavir, and estrogen products such as Premarin® tend to raise blood glucose through intrinsic effects.

63. B: Biguanides and thiazolidinediones (TZDs) are generally contraindicated for those patients with CHF. The use of metformin increases the risk for lactic acidosis. Use of TZDs may lead to fluid and sodium retention. Other classes of medications, including DPP-4 inhibitors, alphaglucosidase inhibitors, sulfonylureas, meglitinides, GLP-1 receptor agonists, and amylin analogs are not summarily contraindicated for use with CHF, but may need to be adjusted and carefully monitored, according to manufacturers' indications.

64. B: Asking open-ended questions to help the patient identify immediate strategies will directly address the patient's desire to accomplish his long-term goal. He has expressed his willingness to make changes. He has already defined the main problem, identified feelings, and set a long-term goal. The next step is to identify short-term goals that will contribute to the realization of the long-term goal. Patient empowerment models of care affirm that ideas and choices generated by patients will have the greatest effect on metabolic control. Choice (A) is redundant since the patient is already aware and convinced that he needs to lower his HbA1c to minimize his risks. Choice (C) is not a bad option but is a goal that comes from the educator, not the patient. If given the chance, the patient might suggest the same strategy. If he doesn't, it is likely not something he is prepared to do. Choice (D) does not address what the patient wants help with right now. His goal is to lower his A1c, not reduce stress level at work. Of course this topic is a worthwhile discussion, but right now you should focus on the immediate concern of the patient.

65. D: The key to management of both acute and chronic sensorimotor diabetic neuropathies is blood glucose control and stability. Several observational studies suggest that neuropathic symptoms improve not only with optimization of control but also with the avoidance of extreme blood glucose fluctuations. Many patients will require pharmacological treatment for painful symptoms. Several medications, including tricyclic antidepressants (amitriptyline), anticonvulsants (gabapentin), SSRIs, and opioids (tramadol) have shown some success in managing symptoms; referral to pain management is also recommended in some cases. Appropriate diagnosis is through clinical findings, including pinprick, temperature, and vibration perception (using a 128-Hz tuning fork), 10-g monofilament pressure sensation at the distal halluces, and ankle reflexes, as well as the exclusion of non-diabetic causes. Consideration of non-diabetic causes might typically include serum B12, thyroid function, blood urea nitrogen, and serum creatinine. This is part of the assessment and diagnosis process, however, and would not be considered key to the management

of sensorimotor neuropathies. Finally, graded supervised aerobic exercise is recommended for those with cardiovascular autonomic neuropathy (CAN).

66. B: Because celiac disease is an immune-mediated disorder, there is a greater prevalence among those with type 1 diabetes, as compared to the general population (1–16% of individuals compared with 0.3–1% in the general population). It is not associated with insulin resistance and not more prevalent among the type 2 diabetes population. Gluten-free diets are not generally recommended as a meal plan option for those who have not been diagnosed with celiac disease, as whole grains provide energy, fiber, and other important nutrients. Screening for celiac disease is recommended for all those with type 1 diabetes, shortly after diagnosis, but *not* for those with type 2 diabetes in the absence of symptoms.

67. A: Steroid effects on glucose metabolism include down-regulation of glucose transporter 4 (GLUT-4) in the muscle so that more insulin is needed for the uptake of glucose into cells. This results in hyperglycemia, specifically post–prandial hyperglycemia. Steroids do not decrease metabolism of insulin and do not increase risk for hypoglycemia. Steroids may also promote glucose production in the liver, reduce binding of insulin to the insulin receptor cells, and decrease insulin secretion from the islet cells, all of which may affect fasting glucose levels, but this is not the most pronounced effect. While steroids do suppress the immune system, it is inaccurate to say that steroids "deactivate" insulin.

68. B: A low-interest medical loan from her local bank would be the *least* helpful option on the list for this patient. The patient's budget is already stretched thin and a loan, even a low-interest loan, would add an extra cost burden. Also, when the loan money runs out, she will likely require the same or greater resources for her medications. The first thing to do would be to see if anything can be done to reduce her cost burden from the perspective of requirements. For example, is it possible that a different testing regimen (one requiring fewer tests per day) may work? Can she use a generic meter that uses less expensive test strips? Once all regimen options have been exhausted, the patient might check with programs and organizations that help those in need, specifically those who are uninsured with low income. Such organizations include Partnership for Prescription Assistance, local and state health department programs, and Needymeds.

69. B: The ADA Standards of Care for Diabetes (2013) state: Patients with prediabetes "should be referred to an effective ongoing support program targeting weight loss of 7% of body weight and increasing physical activity to at least 150 min/week of moderate activity such as walking". While other weight loss goals may be applicable or desired by some patients, the ADA target recommendations are based on results of the DPP, which found that 7% body weight reduction target and increased physical activity resulted in 58% less conversion to diabetes at 3 three years and 34% at 10 years, without medication.

70. B: The development and progression of diabetic retinopathy correlate strongly with both blood pressure and blood glucose control. These risk factors are both modifiable. The risk factor most closely associated with diabetic retinopathy is duration of diabetes. Other modifiable risk factors (although not as heavily correlated) include lipid control and smoking status. Some possible risk factors may include age, glucose variability, clotting factors, renal disease, and use of specific medications, although these factors remain in question.

71. D: There is no specific mix of macronutrients recommended by the ADA. The best mix of macronutrients depends on individual circumstances. Studies thus far have not conclusively identified an optimal mix of macronutrients. Dietary Reference Intakes (DRIs) may be helpful for

patients seeking guidance on an appropriate mix. Regardless of macronutrient mix, total caloric intake must be appropriate to the weight management goals. Option (A) suggests a higher proportion of carbs than typically recommended. Option (B) suggests a higher proportion of protein (and less fat) than typically recommended; this mix is the closest to the dietary reference intakes. Option (C) suggests a lower proportion of carbohydrates than what is normally recommended.

72. C: A reduced-calorie, reduced-fat diet is the primary recommended dietary strategy for those with prediabetes. Not only has this strategy been shown effective at modest weight loss, but the reduction in fat may also improve insulin sensitivity. Low-carb diets for the primary prevention of diabetes are not recommended at this time. Carbohydrate monitoring is a strategy that is recommended for persons with diabetes but not at this time for those with prediabetes. Glycemic index/glycemic load strategies remain unproven at this time and are not recommended as a diabetes prevention strategy.

73. B: Fifteen grapes contain about 15 grams of carbohydrate and no significant protein or fat. When treating hypoglycemia (i.e. 58 mg/dL), a person should consume about 15 grams of carbohydrate that is *not* mixed with fat, for fat will delay the absorption of the carbohydrate. Whole milk, peanut butter, and bread with peanut butter all contain fat that will increase the amount of time it takes glucose to rise.

74. C: By avoiding the area, lipohypertrophy can resolve itself in weeks to months. Therefore, the best advice is to select alternative sites in which to inject insulin. Antibiotic therapy, warm compresses, and surgical removal are not recommended treatment options.

75. A: The patient's social, cultural, and religious preferences should always be accommodated when possible. Several studies have shown that fasting, even with type 1 diabetes, can be accomplished safely. Recommendations include good baseline control, more frequent monitoring, minor adjustment of basal insulin if needed (which is easier with an insulin pump), and prompt treatment of hypoglycemia. Patients in good control do not typically need to reduce basal insulin and should be prepared to end the fast with oral glucose if they experience hypoglycemia. Readdressing the hazards of fasting or talking to the pastor to find an alternative may be perceived as dismissive of the patient's wishes – like trying to "talk the patient out of" the idea. While the patient should be made aware of potential risks, the educator must respect the patient's religious preferences and then present options and information that can help the patient decide on the best course of action.

76. C: While abandoning and revising objectives is part of the goal evaluation process, one must examine reasons why the objective was not achieved. It may be that the patient did not have enough time or that the pace was too aggressive for him, but these are only assumptions until the patient expresses them. It may be that the patient has not identified reasons why physical activity is personally meaningful and he is therefore lacking motivation. At times, it is important to acknowledge successes or ambitions in other self-care areas, rather than dwelling on failures, but without first discussing the physical activity goal in greater depth with the patient, one would not know his desires and obstacles associated with this specific goal. For example, it may be that the patient very much wants to exercise but has not been able to find a safe way to accomplish it.

77. A: According to the National Standards (2013), "it is crucial that the individual with diabetes is viewed as central to the team and that he or she takes an active role." Other persons on the team may include diabetes educators, case managers, and both primary care providers and specialty care

providers such as endocrinologists. Other members of the multidisciplinary team may include nutrition specialists, psychologists and other mental health specialists, physical activity specialists, optometrists, podiatrists, and others.

78. A: "A turkey and cheese, lettuce, and tomato sandwich with an apple, a small serving of baked chips, and a diet soda" is the best example of a *well-balanced* meal. This choice has an appropriate balance of carbohydrate, fat, and protein; the serving sizes are appropriate and fruits and vegetables are included. The sample meals in choices (B) and (C) may be healthy in some ways (low fat, low calorie, etc.), but are not well balanced, as they contain almost no carbohydrate. Conversely, the meal choice in option (D) is almost entirely carbs (with more than 120 grams of carbohydrate).

79. A: Methyldopa is one of the recommended mediations for treating a hypertensive disorder during pregnancy. Other suggested medications include: labetalol, diltiazem, clonidine, and prazosin. This patient meets criteria for preeclampsia: systolic blood pressure ≥140 mmHg or diastolic blood pressure ≥90 mmHg, diagnosed after the 29th week of pregnancy. Preeclampsia must be addressed as safely as possible to prevent maternal and fetal injury. ACE inhibitors and angiotensin receptor blockers (ARBs) are contraindicated in pregnancy. Chronic diuretic use is also not recommended in pregnancy, as it has been associated with restricted maternal plasma volume, which could reduce uteroplacental perfusion. Lifestyle modification should be reinforced, but since the patient has had three blood pressure readings above target and states that she is already following lifestyle recommendations, it is time for the next step.

80. B: In a person who needs 2000 calories per day, the calories from saturated fat should not exceed 140 to 200 calories (or 7% to 10% of total calories). Choice (A) is 2% of total calories and is an unrealistic expectation. Choice (C), which specifies a limit of 200 mg/day for all is referring to dietary cholesterol, rather than calories from saturated fat. Choice (D) specifies a calorie total that represents about 35% of total calories. This is the maximum total calories from fat that is recommended, however, it is untrue that there is no recommendation for saturated fat limit. ADA 2013 Standards of Care recommend no more than 7% of calories from saturated fat. It should be noted that very recently published ADA Nutrition Therapy Recommendations (2013) have modified these recommendations to < 10% of calories from saturated fat to coincide with recommendations for the general population.

81. D: Januvia. Due to the increased creatinine levels, the patient would not be a candidate for metformin, as metformin relies on appropriate kidney function to metabolize appropriately. Metformin use in renal impaired patients may lead to lactic acidosis and is therefore contraindicated for women with serum creatinine above 1.4 mg/dL (> 1.5 mg/dL/min). Likewise, pioglitazone is not a first-line drug and is not recommended for those with CHF. While basal insulin is generally a safe choice, is it not usually used as first-line treatment and the patient is not willing to consider it. Sitagliptin has been shown to be both effective and safe as a first-line diabetes medication and can be used in patients with impaired renal function and history of heart disease, although a reduced dose may be needed.

82. B: A recent evidence-based practice recommendation and an example of translating research into practice is, "unvaccinated adults with diabetes who are aged 19 through 59 years should receive hepatitis B vaccination." For those aged 60 and over, the vaccination may be considered but was not found to be as cost effective. All other options are not current recommendations, according to the 2013 ADA Standards of Care, due to insufficient evidence.

83. C: According to the American Diabetes Association, those with specific co-morbidities should have a thorough medical evaluation. These co-morbidities include proliferative retinopathy or severe non-proliferative retinopathy, as well as autonomic and peripheral neuropathy. An ECG stress test should be performed (especially since the patient is sedentary and has a history of a cardiac issues), as well as an updated retinopathy exam. Adjustments may need to be made to reduce further injury, including no vigorous aerobic exercise or resistance training and possible limitation of weight bearing activities. Beyond cardiac stress testing and retinopathy, additional referrals listed in option (D) are probably not necessary, since she has already been diagnosed and is being managed. A treating physician or other provider should be able to perform the rest of the pre-exercise medical evaluation and help develop an appropriate exercise plan.

84. A: Conversation maps would be the best choice for the above situation for several reasons. Group interaction activities, such as conversation maps, have proven to facilitate learning to a greater extent than passive-learning strategies. In all likelihood, most of the residents can still participate in a discussion-type activity without too much trouble, even with deficits in sight, mobility, or dexterity. A strategy such as this allows those with varying amounts of knowledge/experience to participate equally. Option (B) assumes that all participants will be familiar with how to use laptops. If this proves not to be the case, then you will spend much of your time on computer training. Option (C) might be good to leave for follow-up, but will not yield the learning that discussion does, and participants won't have the option of bringing up their individual concerns. Option (D) does not engage participants and does not allow for much adaptation to the individual needs within the group.

85. B: Web-based activities, role-playing, group discussion, and lecture is a series of appropriate strategies that are ranked in terms of smallest group (individual) to largest. Option (A) is not the best choice because games usually involve more than one person, and demonstration is difficult to do in a large group. Option (C) lists lecture before demonstration; lecture is actually not usually for a small group while demonstration is. Option (D) also lists lecture before printed material. Again, lecture is best used when the group is too large to provide more interaction and printed materials are designed for one person (as reinforcement) rather than group instruction.

86. D: The target for critically ill patients should be between 140 and 180 mg/dL. While lower targets may be appropriate in some cases, targets less than 110 mg/dL are no longer recommended, due to evidence that lower glucose levels resulted in increased mortality among critically ill patients. For non-critically ill patients, the recommended pre-meal target is < 140 mg/dL (not < 100 mg/dL); targets for random BG (non-critically ill) <180 mg/dL (not <140 mg/dL). Again, lower targets may be advisable for certain patients, but targets less than 100 mg/dL are not recommended.

87. B: Cutting back on repaglinide (Prandin®) on mornings she exercises will reduce the amount of insulin released by her pancreas for a short time. With less insulin, she is less likely to experience hypoglycemia, and therefore, she may not need to consume extra glucose after her workouts. To test this, the educator should advise the patient to check glucose before, immediately following exercise, and at periodic intervals afterwards. Advise the patient that she should treat hypoglycemia whenever her glucose drops too low. Consuming a small amount of juice before the activity may prevent the hypoglycemia, but does not address the patient's concern about consuming extra calories. Telling the patient not to worry about the extra calories is dismissive of the patient's values and concerns. Patient-centered care recognizes that patients are likely to adhere to lifestyle modification recommendations when they foresee an outcome that matters to

them. Skipping metformin is unlikely to prevent the hypoglycemia, as metformin does not cause an increase in circulating insulin.

88. A: The HbA1c screening is recommended at least twice annually for patients who meet glycemic guidelines, in this case, less than 7%. The other screenings such as a comprehensive foot exam, dilated eye exam, and fasting lipid profile are indicated once yearly for a patient with these characteristics. Lipid profile may be done every two years for those with very low risk, but since this patient has had borderline LDL levels, the screening should be done annually.

89. D: This patient has answered in the affirmative to depression screening questions. Although you cannot confirm a diagnosis of depression, his answer is sufficient to warrant a referral to a mental health specialist. Depression affects 20 to 25% of the diabetes population (twice that of the general population). Many who suffer from depression with diabetes find adhering to the rigorous self-care activities very difficult, if not impossible. While "burnout" in those with diabetes is not uncommon, his reply to the question indicates it may be something more serious; further evaluation is warranted. Neglect of diabetes self-care will result in poor control, but depression is not something that a person can always "snap out of". He may lack the energy and so the depression must be addressed. Anxiety, on the other hand, is typically characterized by irrational fears and avoidant or extreme behaviors.

90. D: Ketones cross the placenta and are harmful to the fetus, therefore, maternal ketosis should be avoided; thus, option (A) is false. Because ketones represent starvation, when the body must burn fat reserves to meet energy needs, the remedy is usually an increase in dietary intake. However, good blood glucose levels must also be maintained, and therefore the patient will likely need to take insulin with the extra food. Increasing insulin without increased food intake will cause nocturnal hypoglycemia, and adding fat to the diet during the day is not likely to address the patient's needs overnight and may even increase ketosis.

91. C: Of the choices listed, only decreasing lipids has been shown to reduce PAD risks, progression, and/or symptoms. The UKPDS demonstrated that a reduction in blood pressure of 10/5 mmHg (systolic/diastolic) had no effect on the risk of amputation in PAD. As in other atherosclerotic diseases, glycemic control has not been shown to have an effect on the progression of PAD. Only supervised exercise training programs have been shown to be of benefit in improving walking for those with PAD. Unsupervised exercise programs have not yielded such results, nor any of the other results listed in choice (D).

92. D: An avoidant coping style is characterized as doing only the bare minimum and ignoring or blocking additional information that is beyond survival skills alone. Avoidance is often associated with the emotional discomfort that comes with fear, anxiety, anger, shame, or other uncomfortable feelings the patient may be experiencing. An exploration and validation of these feelings should be the priority above reviewing or adding additional diabetes education. Conversely, in the "depression and frustration" emotional stage of chronic disease, a person will often express a loss of control and an inability to handle the expectations associated with diabetes self care. The patient described in this question may have those fears, but has not yet faced them.

93. B: "Changing his insulin-to-carb ratio from 10 to 12 for lunch and dinner only" is the correct option. Because his episodes of low blood glucose do not occur before meals, it is not likely that the basal rate is too high. Likewise, the sensitivity factor would be modified if the patient reported hypoglycemia after correcting for high glucose. Finally, changing the insulin-to-carb ratio from 10

to 8 would actually give the patient more insulin at mealtime, which would likely make the pattern of post-meal hypoglycemia worse.

94. D: None of the patients described require reduced protein diets. Protein intake of 0.8 to 1.0/ kg body wt/day is in the normal range. Pregnant women are recommended protein intakes of 1.1 g/kg/day and so the current intake may actually need to be increased. Similarly, those with serious wounds should have a protein intake of 1.0 to 1.5 g/kg/day. Finally, according to the recently-published 2013 ADA Nutrition Therapy Recommendations, "For people with diabetes and diabetic kidney disease, reducing the amount of dietary protein below the usual intake is not recommended because it does not alter glycemic measures, cardiovascular risk measures, or the course of glomerular filtration rate (GFR) decline."

95. A: The best example of an immediate outcome is one which can be measured at the time of the intervention, in this case, demonstrating proper technique for self monitoring. The other choices are examples of intermediate results over time, indicate behavioral change, and require more than one measurement. Reducing the number of missed doses of medication requires a pre- and post-assessment for comparison to show a reduction. Improvement in HDL is more a clinical indicator than a behavioral objective; the behavior associated with this clinical objective may be to increase exercise, change an element of the diet, or take medication. In addition, it also requires a pre- and post-assessment for comparison. Being 100% compliant on screenings is a goal that would be set that would then require action and is then measured at a later specified date and time. It is an example of an intermediate objective.

96. A: The US Pharmacopoeia, through their Dietary Supplement Verification Program, verifies that the products listed on the label are accurate and pure. The mark does not indicate FDA approval, efficacy, or safety from drug interactions.

97. D: Medical waste disposal laws do indeed vary from state to state, and so patients and educators need to determine specific policies for their respective areas. It is true that in some states (California, for example), sharps must be discarded in official biohazard sharps containers. Likewise, some states (Texas, for example) allow people to put their needles and lancets in a hard plastic container, then tape the lid and throw it away with regular trash. There are a variety of policies that are somewhere in between. A good place to check for the local policy on medical waste disposal is: http://www.safeneedledisposal.org/.

98. A: The staggering of the SMBG profile: before and after meals (rotating meals), can provide data to identify and manage patterns with as few as three to four readings at a given time of day. In two to three weeks, this patient should have four to six readings before and after each meal – enough to potentially see where the problem lies. This pattern will not exceed his allotment of test strips and even leaves him some extras for emergencies such as when his blood sugar feels low or on sick days. Option (B) will offer little insight, especially if his fasting values are close to normal. You would not be able to identify a meal that may be contributing to his high HbA1c. Option (C) is only partially correct. Patients who take insulin do require more frequent self-monitoring, but this patient does not take mealtime insulin (or even mealtime oral meds) at this point. Furthermore, dismissing the financial concern because monitoring is important is not sensitive to the patient's barriers; if he cannot afford the test strips, he may not have a choice.

99. C: The social worker is the team member that is best trained to address issues related to financial, familial, physical, transportation, or social barriers of many kinds. He or she will know of resources or can recommend referral to the necessary specialties for follow-up care. In addition, the

social worker can make recommendations to the prescribing physician based on a focused, thorough assessment of the patient's capabilities and resources.

100. B: The essential outcome of DSME is sufficient knowledge to perform necessary skills and make the lifestyle changes required for satisfactory quality of life. These behavioral changes lead to positive clinical outcomes as well as fewer diabetes-related complications. Decreased healthcare costs are an eventual long-term outcome that comes from improved clinical indicators resulting from positive lifestyle changes.

101. C: When using an insulin pen device, the patient should prime the pen (perform an "air shot") before each use, whereas with a GLP-1 agonist medication, the priming is only done as part of new pen setup (before first use of each pen). Other choices do not accurately reflect the difference between insulin pens and GLP-1 agonist pens. Both pen types require a new pen needle with each use. With both types of medications, the injection site should be rotated. Both medications may be kept at room temperature for the approved in-use time period.

102. A: "Decrease intake of regular soda from three cans to one can per day by Dec. 1" is a *specific* behavioral objective/goal because it stipulates the details of what will be done, including going from what amount to what amount and by what date. Options (B), (C), and (D) all have elements that could be considered ambiguous: what will be done to decrease cardiovascular risk, how will we measure glycemic control, and how will we measure overall health, better eating/rest, and movement, respectively.

103. D: There are many effective ways to track patient progress of behavioral goals, including individual visits, group classes, email or text messaging, phone consultations, regular mail, and other methods. The key is to make sure the method is standardized (i.e. collected consistently at predetermined time points) and convenient for the patient.

104. D: As evidenced by his weight gain and continued high readings, the patient is likely overeating. This is further supported by the fact that occasionally the insulin is sufficient to keep his glucose within target range or even low. The educator should help the patient to evaluate current eating patterns and make adjustments. His BG meter logs may at first indicate a need for more insulin, but the consistent weight gain must also be taken into consideration. Decreasing the dose without addressing the nutritional aspects would leave the patient with high fasting glucose levels. However, once the patient is able to reduce intake, a lower dose of insulin may be needed. At some point, he may also require mealtime insulin, but the weight increase is the first clue that he is overeating; it is best to adjust one element at a time. Bolus insulin would be indicated by BG values that increase consistently after meals throughout the day.

105. A: The Somogyi phenomenon, while rare, is a rebound from hypoglycemia that results in high morning glucose due to an exaggerated counterregulatory response. Dawn phenomenon is elevated fasting glucose in the morning, likely due to overnight growth hormone and increased cortisol. It is not usually preceded by hypoglycemia. The recommendation for those with type 1 diabetes is to adjust insulin to meet appropriate carbohydrate intake. Adding a protein snack at bedtime is not the best approach for this patient; it is questionable whether or not a protein snack would help since protein has not been shown to increase plasma glucose concentrations. In addition, it does not explain why the glucose would "rebound" in the morning after nocturnal hypoglycemia. The "honeymoon period" is a phenomenon that occurs in type 1 diabetes shortly after diagnosis and can last up to 12 months. It is characterized by the need for very little insulin. While the end of the honeymoon period is characterized by greater fluctuation in blood sugars, it would not explain the

consistent pattern of nighttime fluctuations of this patient, especially since he has had diabetes for three years.

106. B: Contemplation, characterized by a person recognizing a problem and potential benefits, yet is hesitant due to concerns over what the change will mean, is the stage of change that best describes this patient. He has stated that he is ready to make minor adjustments if it will help him to achieve his goal. He also qualifies that he wants to learn but is hesitant because he does not see or remember well, and has little perceived control over his food choices. In precontemplation, patients do not yet recognize the problem or the need to make changes. In action, the person is actively engaged in the change process. In maintenance, the person works to sustain the change and help it become habit. None of these last three options apply to Mr. Jones.

107. A: "I will choose items from the restaurant menu that fit with my healthy eating plan, including vegetables, low-fat meat, and 3 servings of carbohydrates" is an appropriate, well-written behavioral objective. Behavioral objectives should begin with an action word: "choose" as opposed to "understand" or "know". In addition, they should reflect the desired behavior, rather than the clinical outcome (i.e. lab values). Finally, they should be customized and meaningful to the patient.

108. C: Open-ended questions that cause the patient to ponder pros and cons of behavior change empower the patient to make those changes based on good understanding. Choice (A) is a redundant and patronizing question. No patient wants to end up on dialysis, therefore the purpose of this type of question is not to gain actual information from the patient or to empower, but rather to warn or badger. Rather than empower, this type of question is likely to make the patient feel childlike and not in control. Furthermore, it is not open-ended; it is inappropriate. Choice (B) is a probing question that might be helpful in assessing the patient's knowledge but does not empower him to make changes. Choice (D) is not the best answer because it did not originate from the patient. While the goals may be appropriate, they are the educator's and not the patient's. Collaboration is important, but empowerment comes from self-identification of challenges, emotions, and solutions that lead to change.

109. D: Printed material from the drug manufacturer regarding the side effects of medications is the least likely to be helpful to Mr. Jones. First, he admits that he has poor near-sight vision and so reading may be difficult. In addition, while printed information is valuable to reinforce instruction, it does not yield the retention of more active teaching methods, including group discussion, hands-on demonstration/return demonstration; or role-playing, whether individually or in a group.

110. A: "Lose ten pounds by October 31 (3 months) by increasing walking to 25 minutes per day and limiting second helpings to just vegetables" is the best example of a behavioral goal for this patient. This goal is measurable (in pounds and in minutes walked), it is realistic and attainable (not too ambitious – less than 1 pound per week), and has a time limit element (3 months). In addition, it is relevant to the patient. He states that he wants to be able to play more golf and play with his grandchildren. Modest weight loss will have a direct impact on his ability to be able to do the things he wants to do. Option (B) does not speak to behavior; it is likely to be a health care provider goal and does not extend to what the patient wants out of life. In addition, 6% A1c may not be appropriate for a man his age in many cases. Option (C) is too vague ("improve my diabetes and overall health) and to all encompassing (doing everything I learned in diabetes class). The same is true for choice (D), which tacks on too many behaviors into one goal. It would be better to work on just one or two behaviors at a time.

111. A: Use of an insulin pen does not need to be addressed in initial DSME; DSME is dynamic and changes as patient needs change. The patient is newly diagnosed and is not starting on insulin. If at six months, he needs insulin, then insulin administration should be discussed at that time. Due to the risk for hypoglycemia with sulfonylureas, a hypoglycemia education should definitely be provided. Likewise, making appropriate food choices applies to anyone with diabetes, even if he claims that he does not have much control over his food since he does not cook. And, preventing diabetes-related complications is important information for anyone with diabetes, regardless of age or health status. Some of the prevention topics should include checking feet daily, having regular eye exams and screening labs, monitoring blood glucose, and many others.

112. D: With small-nerve-fiber neuropathy, which usually presents with pain but without objective signs of nerve damage, the greatest risk is for foot ulceration and subsequent gangrene and amputation. More than 80% of amputations follow a foot injury. About 75% of foot amputations are thought to be preventable. Charcot foot syndrome, increased falls, and decreased mobility are also risks associated with sensorimotor neuropathies, but are not the greatest risks. Cardiac death due to cardiac denervation is the greatest risk associated with diabetic autonomic neuropathy (DAN), and specifically cardiac autonomic neuropathy (CAN).

113. B: Communication among team members is part of standard 7 (individualization) of the National Standards for DSME/S (2013). Proper communication increases the likelihood that all team members will work in collaboration for the patient's benefit. Such practices also reduce duplication of services, which reduces cost, and guide treatment and education-related decisions. While patients are likely to be more satisfied when all team members are working on collaboration, it does not mean that each provider should not perform a thorough assessment pertaining to the purpose for which the patient is seeking treatment or services. HIPAA rules allow for information to be shared among healthcare team members for the purpose of treatment activities without expressed consent from the patient.

114. D: The American Diabetes Association recommends a diagnosis of diabetes be made when a person's HbA1c level is ≥ 6.5% only when "performed using a method that is certified by the NGSP and standardized or traceable to the Diabetes Control and Complications Trial (DCCT) reference assay." In addition, it is recommended that any lab test used to diagnose be repeated to rule out lab error.

115. C: While all of the answers are within the realm of possibility, the most likely explanation is that she is fabricating SMBG values. Four elements, when combined, suggest this explanation. First, the SMBG values and HbA1c are far apart in their correlations. Second, she did not bring her meter (which could be downloaded), but somehow remembered her log book (which is usually kept with the meter). Third, she has every single number filled in; it is highly unlikely that a person would not have missed one test in three months; and fourth, there are no numbers out of target range (highly unusual for anyone with diabetes). This is not uncommon. Even though a patient only hurts herself by lying, many patients fear being lectured or letting down the provider/educator. The best way to avoid this is to establish a trusting, non-judgmental relationship with your patient from the beginning. Anemia and most hemoglobinopathies normally result in lower HbA1c values than fingerstick values would indicate. While no BG meter claims to be 100% accurate, the International Organization for Standardization (ISO) requires that 95% of readings to be ±20% of actual value; this variation would not explain the discrepancy between in-target SMBG results and an A1c of 9.6%. Technique should be evaluated, but again, it is highly unlikely that any technique flaw could be responsible for such a discrepancy.

116. B: Omitting breakfast has *not* been shown to result in weight loss. Having more frequent but smaller meals has been shown to be an effective weight-loss strategy, as has portion control and the use of premeasured meal replacements (liquid meals or prepackaged meals). It is worth noting that reducing overall energy intake to 500 to 1000 kcal less than that which is needed for weight maintenance has been shown to result in a one to two pound per week weight loss, but it is *not* recommended that this calorie reduction be achieved by skipping breakfast.

117. B: The *first* treatment priority in HHS is rehydration to expand intravascular volume and restore renal perfusion. Often, rehydration alone may cause glucose values to come down somewhat. Glucose values, often extremely high (>600 mg/dL), need to be addressed as well, but as a secondary or tertiary priority. Electrolyte imbalances likewise must be addressed (potassium, sodium, phosphorus, magnesium) but come after rehydration in terms of priority. Often, there is an underlying condition, such as infection that precipitates HHS. This must be addressed to prevent relapse, but again, it is not as critical as rehydrating the patient.

118. D: It is accurate to say that the ADA recommends that the HbA1c test should be performed at least twice annually, and more in some cases. For those who have had medication changes or have not reached the glycemic goal, quarterly tests are recommended. Some patients who require intensive management may need even more frequent testing. All other statements are false. A 7% target is a general recommendation for HbA1c. For those with hypoglycemia unawareness, comorbidities, or age concerns (young children or the elderly), the risk of lower HbA1c outweighs the risks associated with a higher A1c. While it is true that the HbA1c has recently been adopted by the ADA as a valid diagnostic tool, the industry recognizes that there are significant variations in HbA1c results among races as well as in those with anemias and hemoglobinopathies. Similarly, the HbA1c test identified fewer cases of previously undiagnosed diabetes than either the fasting plasma glucose or the 2-hour glucose tolerance test.

119. A: Assessing a patient's mastery of a self-care skill should be accomplished by observing return demonstration. This enables the educator to identify improper technique or areas for improvement. Return demonstration with proper technique should be documented to establish proper evaluation. A verbal explanation of the skill does not allow to educator to witness the skill in action and may not reveal some problem areas, such as visual or dexterity issues. Verbal acknowledgement of understanding is the least valid, as it relies on understanding and mastery as *perceived* by the patient. The person with the skill expertise should evaluate the skill level and offer guidance. Verbal response/acknowledgement would be more appropriate for assessments relating to a patient's values and obstacles (information for which the patient *is* the ultimate authority). A post-education assessment is more appropriate for evaluating knowledge level, but may not necessarily translate into application or tactile skills. An advantage of written assessment tools, particularly pre- and post-education, is that change in knowledge or retention of knowledge can be quantifiably measured.

120. B: Children with diabetes do *not* have higher rates of dental caries *but* they do have more plaque and gingival inflammation, and more teeth with poor gum attachment. Dental care with diabetes is very important but often neglected. Only about 65% of persons with diabetes report seeing a dentist in the previous 12 months. Hyperglycemia contributes to increased periodontal disease and periodontal disease contributes to hyperglycemia and increased insulin resistance. Treatment of dental disease has been shown to improve glycemic control and vice versa. In addition to hyperglycemia, some medications for depression and hypertension (diuretics) frequently used by those with diabetes can also lead to increased dental problems because they contribute to dry mouth.

121. C: High triglyceride levels (hypertriglyceridemia) are most closely associated with low HDL levels. Other choices, including high LDL, high glucose, and small-sized LDL particles are also common to those with type 2 diabetes, and are often seen in patients who also have high triglyceride levels. However, the correlation is not as strong.

122. C: The rate of depression for those with diabetes is about twice that of the general population. The role of the diabetes educator when it comes to depression is to screen when appropriate and assist those who may be depressed in obtaining help from a mental health professional. This may include helping the person with the referral and scheduling the appointment, as those who are depressed may lack the energy to accomplish these tasks. Of course, those who have clinical depression that is not treated will also find it very difficult, if not impossible to perform the many self-care behaviors needed for good diabetes management. It is not within the diabetes educator's scope of practice to diagnose depression. Depression is not the same as stress. It is inaccurate to say that an educator can teach strategies that will prevent clinical depression. While communication with the patient's mental health professional may be helpful in helping the patient with diabetes to learn self-care strategies, it is not the priority intervention.

123. A: Proliferative diabetic retinopathy is characterized by neovascularization (new vessel growth) and/or vitreous or preretinal hemorrhage. Any stage on nonproliferative diabetic retinopathy does not include new vessel growth. Severe nonproliferative retinopathy will have more than twenty intraretinal hemorrhages in each of the four quadrants, definite venous beading in 2 or more quadrants, or prominent intraretinal abnormalities in at least one quadrant (but no neovascularization or prerentinal hemorrhage). Mild nonproliferative retinopathy has microaneurysms only. Moderate nonproliferative retinopathy may have more than just microaneurysms but no signs as significant as with severe nonproliferative retinopathy.

124. A: An AADE position statement on inpatient diabetes management (2012) clearly states that "diabetes-specific discharge planning should begin upon admission and should provide smooth transition from hospital to home." There are several elements of a successful discharge, including patient survival skills education (which can be accomplished without a provider order), gathering all patient supplies, and helping arrange follow up appointments. While some elements may require a provider order or prescriptions, many elements of the plan can and should be worked on as soon as it is known that the patient being admitted has diabetes. While educational activities should ideally be performed when the patient is most ready to learn, many things can be done to make the transition smoother for the patient, such as constructing a list of follow-up appointments or writing out instructions on how to use a monitor, etc. An inpatient diabetes educator can certainly facilitate this discharge planning, but other team members (floor nurse, inpatient dietitian, provider, social worker, patients' family members, etc.) can certainly be involved as well.

125. A: Potassium will almost always need to be given for patient with DKA. Although potassium levels often appear normal or even high, hypokalemia is masked by dehydration. When fluids and insulin are given, potassium levels fall. This can result in heart arrhythmias and eventually death. Serum potassium levels should be checked frequently until stable. Serum phosphate may also be low but research does not support supplementation as oral intake of food can correct this. Sodium bicarbonate is typically low as well (<15 mEq/L) in acidosis, but supplementation is controversial. Serum sodium levels may vary, and low levels are sometimes masked by dehydration, but this level is not as critical or as problematic in DKA as potassium.

126. C: It is true that the risk of complications such as congenital abnormalities and spontaneous abortions decreases if the woman with diabetes has optimal glycemic control at the time of conception. If the HbA1c level is less than 7%, the rates are similar to that of the non-diabetic population. All other choices are untrue. Far less than half of all women with diabetes (one study showed 37%) receive preconception counseling. The first priority of preconception counseling for patients wishing to conceive is glucose control, although achieving healthy pre-pregnancy weight may be a goal as well. Some medications, including statins, are contraindicated in pregnancy. Therefore, preconception counseling should include a careful review of medications and discontinuation of any medications that are teratogenic.

127. D: "When patients have changed their behavior and intend to continue with the change, they need to understand that the old behaviors do not just go away; they 'lie in wait' for an opportunity to return. This requires knowledge of relapse prevention and preparation to deal with the temptation." Techniques that are effective in dealing with temptation and risky behavior (to prevent relapse) include being aware of the risky behavior or situations, having a plan to combat negative thoughts and temptations, and employing effective stress management techniques. Denying that the temptation is still there may prevent the person from avoiding or planning for such occasions; this lack of preparation may contribute to relapse.

128. B: The primary recommendation for those with hypoglycemia unawareness is relaxation of glucose targets. Less stringent targets, resulting in several weeks with no episodes of hypoglycemia, have been demonstrated to improve counter-regulation and awareness to some extent in many patients. More frequent monitoring is also advised, including the use of continuous glucose monitoring systems. However, this recommendation is secondary to preventing hypoglycemia through less stringent glucose targets. Hypoglycemia unawareness is related to deficient counterregulatory hormone release and autonomic responses. Unlike autonomic neuropathy, these conditions are caused by hypoglycemia, rather than hyperglycemia. Therefore, more stringent blood glucose control would not be appropriate.

129. C: "Treat the blood sugar as you would any low blood sugar, and then once it is in the normal range, take your regular dose of insulin and eat your regular meal" is the correct option. Choice (A) is the course patients often take, but not only does this *not* address the immediate need to treat the hypoglycemia, it leads to hyperglycemia later, because the meal consumed still requires insulin. Choice (B) is incorrect for the same reason. In addition, taking insulin after a meal puts a person at risk for hypoglycemia hours later when the food has metabolized but the insulin is still peaking. Choice (D) is incorrect because no one should ever take insulin while experiencing a hypoglycemic reaction. The first priority is always to treat the hypoglycemia.

130. D: Apidra® (insulin glulisine) is classified as rapid-acting insulin. It is designed for mealtime insulin coverage and to correct hyperglycemia. The only other choice that is in this class and designed for these purposes is lispro (Humalog®) insulin. Novolin 70/30 is a mix of NPH and regular (an intermediate and a short-acting insulin). Levemir® (detemir) is a long-acting insulin, which is in the same class as the patient's Lantus® (glargine) insulin. Because her insurance will cover Lantus, there is no need to switch her at this point to detemir. Humulin-N (NPH) is an intermediate-acting insulin. It is very different from Apidra and is not typically recommended for mealtime and correction proposes.

131. B: Although the general ADA recommendation is < 7% HbA1c, higher targets should be set for those patients with "history of severe hypoglycemia, limited life expectancy, advanced microvascular or macrovascular complications, extensive comorbid conditions, and those with

long-standing diabetes in whom the general goal is difficult to attain." In cases such as these, the ADA recommends a target of < 8%. Less than 9.5% may put the patient at discomfort from hyperglycemia and may exacerbate her already debilitating complications. More aggressive targets (< 6.5%) may be appropriate for patients "with short duration of diabetes, long life expectancy, and no significant CVD" according to 2013 ADA Standards of Care. To set a target this low would increase the patient's chances of a fatal cardiac event.

132. A: "Some published studies comparing lower levels of carbohydrate intake (ranging from 21 g daily up to 40% of daily energy intake) to higher carbohydrate intake levels indicated improved markers of glycemic control and insulin sensitivity with lower carbohydrate intakes. However, four randomized, controlled trials indicated no significant difference in glycemic markers with a lower-carbohydrate diet compared with higher carbohydrate intake levels." In addition, several trials resulted in improvements in lipid levels, but many trials also suffered from low retention. Safety of low-carb, high-protein diets for those with renal dysfunction is not known and should therefore not be recommended.

133. C: Stress on the body usually results in an increase in hepatic glucose, thereby raising blood glucose levels. All other options will lower blood glucose. Alcohol can cause a drop in blood glucose because, while the liver is metabolizing alcohol, it does not release as much glucose. Alcohol may raise blood glucose if the alcoholic beverage also contains substantial carbohydrates. Those at risk for hypoglycemia are encouraged to eat whenever they consume alcohol.

134. B: When a group member asks a question that is "off topic", the best approach is to answer briefly and then redirect back to the topic at hand. Adult learning principles state that persons learn best when there is something they want to know. These "teachable moments" are a great opportunity to provide information that will be meaningful and memorable. However, it would not be appropriate to completely switch the curriculum plan based on one question. Others in the group may want to know about the material in session 1, and it is likely that session material is meant to build on what was presented previously. Alternatively, it would be dismissive to bypass answering at all; DSME should be individualized, which means providing each individual with the knowledge they seek; therefore options (C) and (D) are not the best choices either.

135. D: Anxiety is manifested by taking extreme measures to avoid a feared outcome. In this case, the patient is cutting her medication, eating ice cream, and avoiding morning blood sugar as ways to deal with her anxiety over nocturnal hypoglycemia. Depression is usually associated with patients stating that they feel down and have a lack of interest or energy to do the things they need to. Eating disorders are mental health concerns, but his patient does not display the typical signs of an eating disorder. She has stated no weight obsessions or body image issues and she admitted that she eats ice cream every night and tells why she does it. While eating the ice cream is not recommended for her with high morning blood sugars, her rationale (that she does not want a low blood sugar) is sound. Denial is an emotional stage (not so much a mental health issue) that is characterized by the patient refusing to admit that there is a problem and therefore taking no steps to address one. Clearly, this patient senses a problem and is actually going farther than she should to address it.

136. A: *Reduced* fiber intake is suggested for patients who suffer from gastroparesis. Other recommendations include: frequent small meals, decreased fat intake, and soft or liquid meals. Vegetables, for example, may still be included in the meal plan, but should be cooked until very soft to aid digestion. Therefore, options (B) through (D) are appropriate modifications and not the correct choices.

137. A: A lipid profile, or cholesterol testing, should be performed when the patient is in a fasting state because recently consumed food can affect the triglyceride level. An advantage of the HbA1c test is that it is not affected by recent food or drink. Urine microalbumin checks the urine for protein and is a screening test for renal impairment. It can be performed randomly, with no fasting required. ALT/AST are parts of a liver function test. Some providers may order this test fasting, because some foods, medications, or alcohol may affect the test. However, this it is not typically necessary.

138. B: According to the ADA National Standards for Diabetes Self Management & Support (2013), "evidence suggests that the development of standardized procedures for documentation, training health professionals to document appropriately, and the use of structured standardized forms based on current practice guidelines can improve documentation and may ultimately improve quality of care." While these documentation and practices may facilitate smoother clinic operations and reduce administrative costs, this is not the reason for the ADA recommendation. It is not true that such practices and attributes are required by the Joint Commission or by insurance carriers.

139. C: "Choices that have the greatest effect on diabetes outcomes are made by patients, not healthcare professionals" is a guiding principle of patient empowerment approaches to DSME/DSMS. Patient empowerment approaches also stipulate that patients are in control of their own self-management, and that the consequences of those choices rest first and foremost on the patient. Option (A) is not a tenant of any DSME theoretical approach, as support (family, healthcare team, peers, etc.) is recognized as a crucial element. Option (B) is a characteristic of the Social Cognitive Theory. Option (D) is a tenant of the Theory of Reasoned Action/Planned Behavior. The latter two theories are examples of traditional theoretical approaches to behavior change.

140. C: LADA, a form of slow-onset type 1 diabetes is the most likely diagnosis for this patient. It is characterized by positive GAD/islet-cell antibodies, a normal to low C-peptide level, and can often be managed with diet in the beginning months or years. Those with this type of diabetes are typically well into their adult years (over age 35) and not usually overweight (although may be). Type 2 diabetes is not the best choice because the patient does not exhibit typically obvious signs of insulin resistance, such as excess weight and family history. In addition, persons with newly diagnosed type 2 diabetes often have a high C-peptide level and do not have positive GAD/islet cell antibodies. Type 1 diabetes is only correct if you categorize LADA as a form of type 1 diabetes, which some organizations do. However, this patient is older than is typical, and maintains an A1c of 6.4 without insulin, even 2 years after diagnosis, so clearly there is a distinction. MODY typically occurs in persons under the age of 25 years (although can also occur in those much older). This is a type of diabetes in which a single genetic defect causes a problem with the pancreas reacting to increasing glucose appropriately. Therefore, it is highly genetic and C-peptide levels may be normal (since endogenous basal insulin is not necessarily affected). Like type 2 diabetes, positive antibodies are not found. Unlike type 2 diabetes, those with MODY are usually not obese and are usually quite sensitive to insulin or sulfonylurea medications.

141. C: Approximately 75 grams of CHO are consumed when the patient eats half the box of this product. There are three serving per box; therefore, half the box would be equivalent to 1.5 servings. Carbohydrates listed on the label are per serving, so 51 times 1.5 is about 75 g of carbohydrate.

142. D: The conclusion that is *not* applicable in this situation is that the patient has correct assumptions about this food. All other answer choices *are* correct assumptions. The fiber in this

food is not high enough to discount from total carbs. The sugars are not as important as the total carbs, nor is the glycemic ranking (i.e. glycemic index) of carbs. These are all common mistakes patients make when interpreting nutritional information on product packaging.

143. D: Patients who take basal insulin should not omit their dose if they are fasting before surgery. Omitting basal insulin will result in high blood glucose before, during, and after surgery, which can lead to surgical site infections. Metformin should be omitted, as taking it on an empty stomach can cause gastrointestinal upset; in addition, any situation that may result in a use of contrast dye, tissue hypoperfusion, or acute renal dysfunction (such as surgery) warrants holding the dose of metformin. Sulfonylurea medications should be omitted as they may cause a drop in glucose due to the mechanism of action on the pancreas. Short-acting insulin should be omitted as well (unless given by the surgical team to correct a high pre-operative glucose), as it is meant to be taken with food and could cause hypoglycemia in someone who is not eating.

144. A: Routine foot soaks should be avoided unless directed by a physician. Moisturizing dry skin (except between toes), washing and drying feet, and trimming long toenails straight across are all appropriate recommendations. Keep in mind that those with poor vision, unsteady hands, neuropathy, and current lower extremity problems may be advised to have a professional trim their toenails. Other foot care recommendations include: check all areas of the feet every day for wounds or signs of infection, inspect shoes for wear and tear and proper fit, avoid going barefoot, test water temperature before stepping into a tub, have regular foot exams, and seek medical care immediately for any potential problems.

145. D: Recent changes to the guidelines reflect evidence of the ACCORD and ADVANCE clinical trials as well as other cardiovascular research data. These data suggest that lower systolic blood pressure levels (120 mmHg and less) are not beneficial at preventing cardiovascular events. Option (A) is lower than the recommended systolic target; options (B) and (C) list a diastolic of 90 mmHg, which is higher than recommended.

146. C: The best choice of an example of individualization of "make better food choices" is "switch to diet soda and sugar-free ice cream." Individualizing can be accomplished by asking a patient, "What specifically does this statement mean to you?" Making better choices to reduce HbA1c may describe the ultimate purpose for the behavioral goal, just as "over the next six months" specifies the time-specific aspect, but they do not speak to what "making better food choices" will mean to the patient's current eating routine. Reporting to the educator is a good example of breaking the goal down and helping the patient to be accountable, but again, it does not describe the behavioral goal in personal terms. Goals should be individualized so that the patient knows just what actions to take. Furthermore, individualized goals should be documented in the most patient-specific terms to facilitate adjustment to the education and plan of care, communication between healthcare team members, and to demonstrate adherence to the guidelines.

147. B: The evidence for a treatment effect of sleep apnea on glycemic control is mixed and inconclusive. Sleep apnea can be life threatening and is a risk factor for cardiovascular disease. Treatment of sleep apnea significantly improves quality of life and blood pressure control. It is true that persons who are obese, particularly those with central adiposity, are four to ten times more likely to have obstructive sleep apnea. In fact, the rate of sleep apnea in obese participants enrolled in the Look AHEAD trial exceeded 80%. It is estimated that the prevalence in general populations with type 2 diabetes may be up to 23%.

148. A: Restriction of foods high in vitamin K, such as leafy green vegetables, is advised for those on warfarin (Coumadin®) therapy, due to the effect on clotting mechanisms. It does not pertain to those with CKD. General recommendations for those with mild to moderate CKD include good glycemic control, strict blood pressure control with an ACE inhibitor or ARB, and abstaining from NSAIDs. Other recommendations include optimal glycemic control, insulin adjustment as needed to prevent hypoglycemia due to longer action time, and treatment for anemia and osteodystrophy that often accompany CKD.

149. D: The 2008 study (with 2011 follow-up) found no connection between duration of diabetes and the likelihood to restrict insulin. Restrictors were more likely to be younger, had higher HbA1c values, and reported lower self-care scores and higher levels of diabetes-specific stress. During the initial 11-year study period, those women who restricted insulin were more than three times more likely to die (age of death 45 vs. 58 years) and had increased rates of DKA and some diabetes-related complications.

150. D: Acesulfame-K, aspartame, Neotame, saccharin, sucralose, and Stevia have all been shown to be safe, and are approved for use even during pregnancy/breastfeeding, according to the FDA. There is no contraindication for pregnant/breastfeeding women for aspartame, saccharin, Neotame, or any others of the approved nonnutritive sweeteners. However, Stevia was approved fairly recently (Dec. 2008), and there is little specific research on the use of Stevia during pregnancy.

151. A: All of the options are prerequisites for CSII therapy *except* a diagnosis of type 1 diabetes. Candidates for CSII must be insulin requiring, with little to no endogenous insulin production, but there are many patients with type 2 diabetes who also meet this criteria. Patients should be proficient at counting carbohydrates, as the pump delivers bolus doses based on the carbohydrate information entered by the patient. Clinical indications, as recommended by the ADA and AADE, include failure to obtain optimal glycemic control on multiple daily injections of insulin. Also, the patient should demonstrate motivation and consistent blood glucose monitoring. Other prerequisites include being able to calculate bolus insulin doses and having good problem solving skills. In addition to these prerequisites, other skills will need to be mastered before pump therapy is initiated.

152. A: Providing proof of services rendered by the educator, for use to justify practice hours for certification is *not* listed as a purpose of documentation of a patient's assessment, education plan, and documentation in the ADA National Standards for Diabetes Self Management & Support. "Documentation of participant encounters will guide the education process, provide evidence of communication among instructional staff and other members of the participant's health care team, prevent duplication of services, and demonstrate adherence to guidelines."

153. B: The patient's sample meal has close to 60 grams of carbohydrate. The amount of carbohydrate in bread can vary by quite a bit; however, 15 grams per slice can be used for a rough estimate. In addition, $\frac{1}{2}$ a grapefruit is also estimated at 15 grams. One cup of milk has approx. 12 grams of carbohydrate. Added together, this is reasonably close to 60 grams. A person that is counting carb servings (estimated at 15 grams per serving) would count 4 servings for a total of 60 grams. If someone needed an exact amount, he or she would need to consult bread labels, measure the milk, etc. Some patients may be advised (or may prefer) to count exact carbs, but many will estimate and can benefit from practice from estimation exercises.

154. A: If adults with diabetes choose to use alcohol, they should limit intake to a moderate amount (one drink per day or less for adult women and two drinks per day or less for adult men), according to the ADA 2013 Standards of Care. Choice (B) is more alcohol than the recommended limit for persons with diabetes. Option (C) is incorrect because persons with diabetes may consume alcohol in moderation, although they should take precautions to prevent hypoglycemia, such as eating food if taking insulin or using sulfonylurea medications. Option (D) is also incorrect, as it includes the words "without restriction," implying that any amount is acceptable.

155. D: According to American Diabetes Association Standards of Care (2013), patients with blood pressure greater than 120/80 mmHg should be advised on lifestyle changes to reduce blood pressure. Patients with confirmed blood pressure ≥ 140/80 mmHg should "have prompt initiation and timely subsequent titration of pharmacological therapy to achieve blood pressure goals". People with diabetes should be treated to a blood pressure of <140/80 mmHg, but some persons (such as younger patients) may benefit from lower targets, such as 130/80 mmHg. Choice (A), ≥150/90 mmHg, is higher than the indicated threshold for hypertensive pharmacological treatment and much higher than the recommended threshold of 120/80 mmHg lifestyle change recommendations.

156. D: RPE is a subjective rating in which the patient estimates the exertion level based on feelings of exertion and fatigue. The original scale rates perceived intensity from 6 to 20, with moderate/vigorous-intensity equating to a 12 to 16 on the scale. Choices (A) and (C) are not actual intensity estimation tools. If these were tools, they would not be "perceived" since the estimate would be on actual measurements. An actual method that is similar is the heart rate reserve (HHR), which uses a formula to calculate 55 to 90 percent of the maximum heart rate. This method can be very confusing for those with limited literacy/numeracy abilities. Choice (B) actually describes the "talk test", which would be another appropriate intensity estimation method to use with this patient.

157. C: Medications are the specialty of pharmacists. They are trained to consider the dose, timing, drug interactions, side effects, and contraindications of all prescription medications, including those for diseases other than diabetes, as well as over-the-counter drugs and supplements, such as vitamins. If this patient has a healthcare team with an assigned pharmacist, then the pharmacist would be the best person to address this patient's medication-related concerns. That team member can then communicate any problems with the regimen to the rest of the team. Most likely, many providers have prescribed medications in this patient's regimen, which would make it difficult to address all of her concerns at once. Without a physical complaint or a follow-up, an "education" appointment may be difficult to have covered by insurance. A mental health visit is not indicated either, as her concerns are very appropriate under the circumstances and no anxiety treatment is likely necessary. While a RD/CDE is likely informed about the diabetes regimen medications, he or she may not be able to answer all questions about how they interact with the medications for the other conditions. If the concern were primarily dietary, then this may be the best choice. However, other team members should be made aware of the patient's concerns as well as any changes made to the regimen.

158. C: "Run 20 minutes at least 3 times per week" can be measured by the patient, both in terms of minutes per run and number of runs per week. To achieve goals, patients need to be able to track progress in a measureable way. Choice (B) is not stated in a way in which the achievement can be measured. It could be re-written to be measurable, though, by including minutes on a treadmill or number of miles run. Similarly, Choice (A), "improve diabetes control by managing my portion size," needs to be specified in terms that can be measured (no more than 60 grams of carbohydrate per

meal, etc.), as does choice (D), "keeping my ophthalmology appointments," which should include information such as how many appointments or how often.

159. A: Commencement, which involves determining when the exercise plan should start, is not part of the standard exercise prescription, although it is important when helping patients set physical activity goals. The five components of an exercise prescription are: mode, which includes what type of activity will be performed, intensity, frequency, duration, and progression. The exercise prescription is a plan the patient follows to improve physical fitness. The challenge for the clinician is "to design a plan that meets the patient's desired fitness goals."

160. B: Backdating the meter to accept expired test strips is *not* an appropriate cost-cutting strategy. Accuracy of results would be suspect and with an incorrect meter date, both the patient and provider may easily become confused when examining data and making regimen changes. Appropriate cost-cutting strategies include using a less expensive generic meter or test strips, testing less frequently but often enough and at the right times so that trends can be seen, and sticking with the brand of meter and strips most covered by the patient's insurance carrier. Sometimes, a clinic staff member will suggest a meter with which they are most comfortable and confident, but patient-centered care considers barriers to the patient and makes accommodations when possible. Anything that will allow the patient to monitor consistently will ultimately be best.

161. A: ADA 2103 Standards of Care states: "Administer pneumococcal polysaccharide vaccine to all diabetic patients >2 years of age. A one-time revaccination is recommended for individuals > 64 years of age previously immunized when they were < 65 years of age if the vaccine was administered > 5 years ago."

162. D: "Walk briskly for 25 minutes every day following dinner" is a behavioral goal that is realistic and attainable for most patients with the above health history. Position statements and ADA recommendations stipulate that 150 minutes (25 minutes X 6 days per week in this case) of moderate intensity, such as brisk walking, is the minimum goal for patients with type 2 diabetes. Option (A) does not come close to the recommended standard and is not likely to stretch this patient's abilities as an attainable goal should. Options (B) and (C) are too aggressive and are not likely achievable for a patient with the characteristics of someone who is sedentary and overweight.

163. C: Of the patients above, only the man with ischemic heart disease who uses a nitrate-containing medication is contraindicated from using PDE5 inhibitor medications. This is due to a potentially serious, even fatal drop in blood pressure that may occur. For mild to moderate kidney disease and liver disease, the dose of the medications may need to be adjusted. For severe hepatic or renal disease, such as for those on dialysis, some of these medications are contraindicated. Check detailed manufacturers' information for details before suggesting to patients.

164. D: Preconception counseling should be provided on a regular basis to every woman of child-bearing age with diabetes. This counsel is particularly important to this patient because she is on her own at school and admits to "slacking" on her diabetes self-management, which may also mean that she is not being as careful in other areas. There is no indication that the patient has undiagnosed kidney problems, especially at a diagnosis duration of three years. Similarly, dilated eye exams are recommended at five years from onset for those with type 1 diabetes. Further MNT (assuming the patient received MNT at diagnosis) is not indicated unless there is some change in health status that warrants a different diet or need for more in-depth education, such as if the patient is preparing for insulin pump therapy. The educator is capable of reviewing dietary principles, including alcohol consumption.

165. C: The most appropriate response to her question about why she should increase her basal rate during a time of illness is to explain that stress increases hepatic glucose production, and therefore, basal insulin needs increase as well. Other choices are incorrect, although each contains a small bit of truth. While insulin dose lowers glucose, extra insulin is needed during times of illness, even if not eating to address increased hepatic glucose. Too little insulin in a person with type 1 diabetes can rapidly lead to diabetic ketoacidosis (DKA). Not taking enough insulin, including on sick days, is a major contributor to DKA. Choice (B) is correct in that food/calories are required for energy needed by the body to fight illness and to prevent DKA, however the purpose of insulin is not that of appetite stimulant. Choice (D) is correct in that drinking at least 8 oz of fluid per hour is recommended, but the recommended increase in basal insulin is not due to poor absorption, but rather increased demand.

166. C: The ADA states "Bariatric surgery may be considered for adults with BMI ≥ 35 kg/m² and type 2 diabetes, especially if the diabetes or associated comorbidities are difficult to control with lifestyle and pharmacological therapy" (2013). Patients should first try other methods, but even if unsuccessful, bariatric surgery is not warranted unless the patient's BMI is 35 or greater. Similarly, it is not a recommended option at this time even for dangerous comorbidities if the patient's BMI is less than 35. Although small trials have shown glycemic benefits of bariatric surgery in patients with type 2 diabetes and BMI 30–35 kg/m², the ADA finds there is currently insufficient evidence to generally recommend surgery in patients with BMI less than 35 kg/m² outside of a research protocol.

167. D: To accurately assess what patients are taking, as well as their understanding and habits of medication administration, it is best to have patients bring all medications in original containers and describe what each is for, when they take it, and any problems they experience. This allows the educator to get a sense of their medication knowledge and health literacy, and allows the educator to check prescription dates and other details. A written medication quiz will not give you all the information you need, including an idea of patient habits, and would not be valid if the patient has a literacy deficit (which in and of itself can contribute to non-adherence). Similarly, studying the chart notes and comparing written lists may provide pieces of the picture but leave out important parts that reflect the patient's own experience and challenges.

168. C: Patients are usually instructed to use the sides of the fingers because there tends to be less pain, due to fewer nerve endings. All other options are false. There is no evidence to date that it is easier to obtain a drop of blood from the side than from the tip of the finger due to better blood circulation. Patients should clean their hands thoroughly, so germs are not the reason for this advice. Blood from the fingertips or the sides of the fingertip is equally representative of whole blood. Some sites, such as the arm and leg may not represent the true value as well. Keep in mind that while the side of the finger is suggested, if a patient prefers to lance the tip of the finger instead, the educator should accommodate his or her preferences.

169. C: SGLT2 inhibitors, such as canagliflozin (Invokana®) work by preventing the reabsorption of glucose in the kidneys. The result is that more sugar leaves the body through the urine and less stays in the bloodstream. Because the mechanism of action is dependent on normal (or close to normal) renal function, this class of medications is contraindicated for those with severe kidney disease (<30 ml/min or on dialysis). Sulfonylurea medications work on the pancreas to release more insulin into the bloodstream. Because the action of endogenous insulin is prolonged with decreased kidney function, the dose may need to be adjusted or even discontinued for those with renal impairment. Biguanides work primarily by reducing hepatic glucose. Because biguanide

medications are broken down by the kidneys, they are contraindicated for those with renal impairment. Use of biguanides with renal impairment may result in excess of the medication in the body, which could result in lactic acidosis. DPP-4 inhibitors may be used with renal impairment, but a reduced dose may be needed, depending on the degree of renal impairment.

170. B: Risk of severe hypoglycemia *increases* with age due to slower metabolism of insulin and other medications. Therefore, older adults will typically see a reduction in the needed dose as age advances. Reduced metabolic rate, altered pain perception, and deceased renal function are all age-related physiologic changes that may require adjustments to the patient's diabetes treatment plan. Other concerns include decreased appetite, sense of taste and smell, higher risk for falls and fractures, memory and cognitive deficits, and others.

171. A: While snacks are important, they should contain carbohydrates in case of low blood sugar or a delayed meal. Snacks such as nuts and cheese may be helpful if a person gets the "munchies" but for safety, he should bring hard candy, fruit, or some other form of carbohydrate. All other items listed should be included in carry-on baggage when traveling.

172. D: The proper use of the blood glucose meter along with a personalized monitoring schedule would be the priority item to discuss at the visit. Mrs. M. has already expressed concern that she is not sure if she is using the meter correctly and that she is not sure when she would test. She has demonstrated that she is willing to monitor by her actions, and is ready for guidance in this area. Discussing diabetes-related complications is too broad and potentially overwhelming for a first discussion. Because the patient has not questioned the meaning of her A1c results, it is a topic that could be reserved for comprehensive diabetes education at a later time. Insulin administration does not apply to this patient at this time.

173. A: Based on the given information, group diabetes self-management education makes the most sense. Education plans should be individualized. While any of the first three options are valid ways to provide diabetes education, Mrs. M is a "sociable" person, and does not have any conditions or characteristics that would warrant one-on-one education. Group education is cost effective, and also allows for interaction with group members as well as the educator, unlike printed information. In addition, research shows that group education can be just as satisfying and clinically effective as one-on-one education, if not more so.

174. B: The patient has admitted that she misses her evening dose of metformin about half the time. Reducing the number of missed doses is a goal that targets a specific behavior – taking medication. The educator can help her devise ways to remember to take her medication and set up a plan for reporting her progress. In addition, it is a goal that is not overwhelming. Other options, such as losing 10 pounds, reducing A1c, and reducing the risk of complications are outcomes that come from achieving specific behavioral goals, such as reducing portion sizes, taking medication more consistently, scheduling appropriate screening appointments, walking 150 minutes per week, etc.

175. C: A referral to a registered dietitian for medical nutrition therapy is recommended as a standard of care for all persons with diabetes. The American Diabetes Association (2013) states: "Individuals who have prediabetes or diabetes should receive individualized medical nutrition therapy (MNT) as needed to achieve treatment goals, preferably provided by a registered dietitian familiar with the components of diabetes MNT". It is recommended that this referral be made as part of the comprehensive diabetes evaluation. In additional to being a recommended standard of care for all, MNT is particularly appropriate for this patient because she is overweight and has expressed concern about changes to her diet. A dilated eye exam with an ophthalmologist is

definitely warranted because she has been diagnosed with type 2 diabetes, but the patient has already scheduled a retinal exam. Finally, mental health referral at this point is premature. Mrs. M.'s reactions and concerns are normal and expected. There is no indication that her psychological state is interfering with her abilities to learn about her diabetes or perform self-care activities. However, it would be wise to conduct a depression screening at this and future visits, especially if she exhibits signs that her mental and psychological health are suffering.

176. A: The American Diabetes Association recommends cholesterol goals of: LDL < 100 mg/dL, HDL > 40 mg/dL (men) and > 50 mg/dL (women), triglycerides < 150 mg/dL. In option (B), both LDL and triglyceride targets listed are too high. Option (C) focuses on total cholesterol, which is not emphasized as much as LDL; it omits LDL, which is the primary target, and also does not differentiate between men and women for HDL goals. Option (D) has mixed up the LDL and triglyceride goals as well as the men's and women's targets for HDL.

177. D: Under current Medicare guidelines, only the treating physician can refer patients for medical nutrition therapy. Medicare will not accept a referral from a CDE, pharmacist, or qualified non-physician practitioner. Typically, Medicare covers three hours of MNT in the first year of diagnosis with 2 hours per year in each subsequent year. This benefit is different from diabetes self-management training (DSMT), the referral for which may be made by a physician or a qualified non-physician practitioner. DSMT and separate MNT services may not be provided or billed on the same day but may be performed by the same person (if the CDE is an RD) on separate days. While Medicare and other insurance providers' coverage can be a detailed and confusing system to navigate, it is important to assist the patient by making sure referrals are provided in a manner that provides maximum reimbursement to the patient. See references for more information on Medicare reimbursement.

178. A: Weight is a modifiable risk factor for diabetes. While family history, race, and age are risk factors for type 2 diabetes, they are not considered modifiable. Physical activity is another modifiable risk factor.

179. C: The key question that people involved in the role of social support should ask themselves is, "What does the person with diabetes want in the way of support?" The person with diabetes should verbalize his or her support needs clearly, and may require educator "coaching" to become comfortable with this. Sometimes well-meaning friends and family can be overbearing, which not only strains the relationship, but also does not usually result in improvement for the person with diabetes. By contrast, some family and friends may be disengaged or distant when it comes to supporting their loved one with diabetes. This can be frustrating for the person with diabetes who may benefit from help from the educator in finding ways to involve loved ones to an extent that is both helpful and comfortable for all those involved.

180. B: Serum creatinine is used to calculate glomerular filtration rate (GFR), a measure of kidney function. Any level above 1.3 mg/dL for men or 1.1 mg/dL for women is considered out of normal range and should be examined further. A serum creatinine of 3.6 mg/dL for a woman would translate to a GFR of 20% for an African-American woman and 16% for those of other ethnicities, if using the MDRD formula. This would equate to stage 4 CKD. Therefore, this statement is true. Statement (A) is false because someone with HDL of 30 mg/dL is still at risk for CVD, even with total cholesterol of less than 200 mg/dL. Statement (C) is false because an HbA1c of 5.9% may be the result of many lows and some high glucose levels, just as it may indicate good control. The SMBG values are needed to determine this. Statement (D) is false because creatinine is a measure of kidney function, not liver function. Liver function tests include ALT, AST, and alkaline phosphatase,

among others. Less than 56 IU/L is the normal range for ALT, but still does not rule out fatty liver disease.

181. C: Optimism is the attribute studied most extensively in terms of healthy adaptation to diabetes; it has proven to positively affect behavioral change. Other common characteristics of those who adapt well to stressors, such as with a chronic disease, are strong internal resources, a sense of purpose, high confidence levels, and overall hardiness, although these attributes have not been linked to success to the same extent as a sense of optimism. Stubbornness, affluence, and consistency may be viewed as assets in and of themselves but have not been identified in the literature as attributes common to those who adapt well.

182. B: The main difference between *process evaluation* and *summative evaluation* is in the purpose of each. The purpose of process evaluation is to determine and make needed adjustments to the educational process. The purpose of summative evaluation is to determine the effects or outcomes of education efforts. Both types evaluate the instruction; the educator is evaluating elements of the actual education (from different perspectives), not evaluating a patient. For both types of evaluation, the process involves gathering data, summarizing, interpreting, and making a judgment as to whether or not the action or program being studied was successful or is in need of adjustments. Both can be used to gather data for reports and/or to make changes. The scope of formative evaluation is limited to a learning experience, such as a class or workshop and examines issues such as the appropriateness of timing, materials, logistics, etc. The scope of summative evaluation encompasses the whole education process but focuses on effectiveness in terms of patient learning and behavioral objectives.

183. B: A systematic process is required for effective continuous quality improvement. Once a problem has been identified, the next step is to analyze the data to determine what the root of the problem may be. In this case, the educator made the assumption that participants wanted more information on the mechanisms of action of oral medications. In fact, it may have been that there was too much information, the information was not applicable, the class was too long, or any other number of reasons. Without further analysis, time, effort, and other resources may be spent in the wrong way. There is no indication that incomplete explanation of the idea to the CQI team resulted in poor satisfaction. Likewise, most patient satisfaction tools that simply ask participants to tell you in some way how satisfied they were present an accurate reflection of this metric. Finally, the educator's proposed change may have been the purpose solution for dissatisfaction that resulted from not enough information on mechanism of action. While creativity is very valuable in some circumstances, sometimes the solution can be straightforward if the cause of the problem is clearly identified.

184. D: To make sure that health information is protected in a way that does not interfere with a patient's health care, information can be used and shared (without written permission) with a patient's family, relatives, friends, or others the patient identifies who are involved with his/her health care or health care bills, unless the patient objects. Therefore, options (A) and (B) are incorrect. However, some healthcare organizations have policies that go a step further to secure patient healthcare information, and so it is a good idea to know your organization's policies. Remember that HIPAA stipulates that patients have a right to their healthcare record, including labs. It is dismissive to say that the result is not important and can wait.

185. B: "Limiting the specialized skill of providing evidence-based diabetes education to health care professionals who are certified as diabetes educators" is not an advocacy goal identified by the American Association of Diabetes Educators. In fact, the AADE recognizes five levels of diabetes

educators, only the top two of which are certified as professional diabetes educators. Levels one through three include non-healthcare professionals such as volunteers that may assist with support groups, healthcare professionals not functioning in roles as diabetes educators, and non-credentialed diabetes educators, respectively. Statements (A), (C), and (D) are three of the six advocacy goals. Other goals include: "providing AADE members with tools and resources to stay engaged in public policy and be better equipped to advocate on their own behalf," "supporting programs and initiatives that detect diabetes or serve to prevent more people from developing the disease," and "educating Congress, State legislators, and other professional organizations and stakeholders about AADE's advocacy priorities."

186. C: To reduce the risk of transmitting blood-borne diseases, all efforts should be made to limit any possible contact with another person's blood. In an inpatient setting, it violates infection control recommendations to use the same pen, which will come in contact with patients' skin, and possibly blood, even with a new pen needle. If the educator wants to instruct with a training pen, then he or she should use a new distinct pen each time, and properly discard after use. An alternative to this would be to demonstrate with the pen, injecting into simulated skin, and then have the patient demonstrate injection technique using his or her own pen or a sterile disposable syringe. With regards to other answer choices, soap and water is now preferred over alcohol to prep fingers for blood glucose self-monitoring. Clinics are within infection control guidelines to use one meter to check blood glucose of many patients as long as a sterile, single-use lancet is used for each person. Finally, if parents use a sterile single-use syringe for each child, then withdrawing insulin from the same vial would not violate infection control principles.

187. C: Assessment implies gathering and interpreting data for the purpose of directing action, whereas evaluation is to determine the extent to which an action or process was successful. Both assessment and evaluation can be clinical or non-clinical in nature. While assessment is done in initial stages, it is often performed after interventions, such as to assess a patient's progress towards a goal or assess his or her skill in checking blood glucose. The data gathered will then dictate the next steps the educator might take.

188. B: Reaching out to referring providers is the most reliable source of patients. Although it usually requires an investment of time and effort, it often yields excellent and consistent results, especially once a trusting relationship has been established. Radio ads (as well as print ads, etc.) and word of mouth are also valuable and sometimes effective marketing strategies, but have not been shown to produce as consistent results. Finding previously hospitalized hyperglycemic patients may constitute a HIPAA violation if potential candidates are discovered through accessing protected health information for marketing purposes. Referral to a program by the hospital physician as part of hospital discharge process is of course a valid method to add participants, but also falls under the category of outreach to referring providers.

189. D: November is when National Diabetes Month (or American Diabetes Month) is observed each year. The first National Diabetes Week, which later evolved into National Diabetes Month, was observed in 1948. On its website, the National Diabetes Education Program (a partnership sponsored by the National Institutes of Health and Centers for Disease Control and Prevention), declares that National Diabetes Month, "is a time for individuals, organizations, and communities across the country to shine a spotlight on diabetes." This national annual campaign presents great opportunities for local diabetes education outreach and advocacy activities.

190. A: The ADA National Standards for Diabetes Self-management Education and Support advocate for the "development of action-oriented behavioral goals and objectives". In addition, learning

objectives should be demonstrative, or able to be witnessed. Words like "know" and "understand" are difficult to measure. One would ask, how can we verify that he or she knows or understands? Improving HbA1c is a worthy long-term clinical goal, but does not qualify as a behavioral objective. What action does the patient need to do to result in an improved HbA1c? Those actions would be more appropriate behavioral objectives.

191. B: Models of foods, nutrition labels, and sample restaurant menus would be the most appropriate materials for this class. Copies of the ADA guidelines would not be appropriate because they are written for healthcare professionals, and your audience may contain people with low literacy levels. Likewise, graphs comparing HbA1c with rates of complications may be confusing to those with low literacy or numeracy, and such materials do not address issues of food. Similarly, foot care props do not relate directly to nutrition and would distract from the topic of the lesson. They would however be very appropriate for a class on reducing risk and preventing complications through good foot care.

192. A: Because there are no signs for medication names and many other proper nouns, a sign language interpreter would have to spell out the word each time you spoke it. Writing the name would make it simpler and more efficient for the interpreter because he or she could point to the name. While visual aids, (including pictures) are very helpful for the hard-of-hearing population, there is no reason to eliminate text based on a hearing disability alone. This modification would be more appropriate for those with a literacy deficit. Arranging chairs in a circle would be helpful if all in the group were conversing with each other. In this case, however, all in the group will need a clear view of the ASL interpreter, who will be communicating your words. In a circle, some would be able to see the interpreter, but some would not. Because you have secured an interpreter, there is no essential need for paper and pen. If class members have questions, they can sign the question and the interpreter can ask you and respond in like manner. A paper and pen may be a nice touch for participants to take notes for themselves, but no more so than for a hearing audience.

193. C: Recent survey data found that rural areas, particularly in the southern states, are underserved by diabetes educators. These studies also found that the majority of diabetes education practices (75%) are located in urban or suburban areas, and the majority was in the most highly populous states.

194. D: It is true that tension and disagreement between primary care providers and diabetes educators regarding self-care recommendations has been found to be a barrier to patients' access to diabetes education, according to a national study. This can often be avoided or at least resolved with effective communication. This same study revealed that most physicians want their patients to have more diabetes support and also want patients to have easier access to diabetes education. Patients over the age of 65 have a much higher rate of diabetes than their middle-aged counterparts. However, they are less likely to participate; only one-third of patients seen by diabetes educators were over the age of 65. Similarly, although rates of diabetes are highest among minority populations (Hispanic, African American, Native American, Pacific Islander, etc.), the majority of patients seen by diabetes educators are non-Hispanic whites.

195. C: Responsibilities of a diabetes educator include promoting diabetes advocacy. Contacting the principle, nurse, and district to explain the situation and suggest reasonable options is the best way the educator can advocate for the patient in this case. The American Diabetes Association position statement on Diabetes Care in the Schools and Day Care Setting (2013) states: "Federal laws that protect children with diabetes include Section 504 of the Rehabilitation Act of 1973, the Individuals with Disabilities Education Act, and the Americans with Disabilities Act. Under these laws, it is

illegal for schools and/or day care centers to discriminate against children with disabilities. Any school that receives federal funding or any facility considered open to the public must reasonably accommodate the special needs of children with diabetes. The required accommodations should be documented in a written plan, such as a Section 504 Plan or Individualized Education Program (IEP). The needs of a student with diabetes should be provided for within the child's usual school setting with as little disruption to the school's and the child's routine as possible and allowing the child full participation in all school activities." The position statement goes on to advocate, "if desired by the student and family, the school should provide permission and opportunity for the student to check his or her blood glucose levels and take appropriate action to treat hypoglycemia in the classroom or anywhere the student is in conjunction with a school activity." Other answers would be circumventing the student's rights or would be shirking the advocacy responsibility of a diabetes educator by suggesting the mother handle it all.

196. A: Evaluation is defined as "the systematic process by which the worth or value of something, in the case of DSME, teaching/learning, is judged." This is part of the 5th step in the DSME process: assessment, goal setting, planning, implementation, and evaluation and monitoring.

197. A: The first step toward providing better quality DSME programs is to reflect on the question, "Are the methods used to provide patients with the services they need and want effective?" This is often answered by systematically examining process and outcome data. Once it has been determined that effectiveness is less than it could be, the data should be further analyzed to reveal the root of the problem. Only then should one ask what programs or initiatives might improve effectiveness, followed by what resources will be needed to make the change and how will the effectiveness of change be measured. By considering all of these questions in a systematic way, continuous quality improvement will result in ever-improving delivery of DSME.

198. A: The National Certification Board for Diabetes Educators (NCBDE) does not accredit or recognize programs. Rather, they "promote the interests of diabetes educators and the public at large by granting certification to qualified health professionals involved in teaching persons with diabetes, through establishment of eligibility requirements and development of a written examination." The American Diabetes Association and the American Association of Diabetes Educators both recognize diabetes self-management education programs. Each has a list of specific requirements and stipulations, although they are all similar and both incorporate the National Standards for DSME. Prior to February 2011, Indian Health Services also recognized programs.

199. D: National Standards for Diabetes Self-Management Education and Support (2013) do not specify which outcomes should be tracked. However, it is clarified by the AADE that "Programs must set behavioral goals with their participants in order to evaluate the effectiveness of the education and interventions provided by the program. Programs must also collect clinical outcome measures in order to evaluate the effectiveness of the change in behavior. Programs must have a system in place to collect behavior/clinical outcomes in order to aggregate and evaluate effectiveness of the education and interventions". While other answers may be useful to evaluate effectiveness of a specific program or intervention, they are not ADA or AADE-required aggregate objectives.

200. A: Poor attendance due to a lack of trust was *not* a finding of the study; in fact, lack of trust and other barriers to care were cited as reasons for the prevalence of diabetes health fairs in high-risk population areas. All other statements were indeed findings of researchers who observed and interviewed involved persons at various community-based screenings throughout New York City in 2007.

Secret Key #1 - Time is Your Greatest Enemy

Pace Yourself

Wear a watch. At the beginning of the test, check the time (or start a chronometer on your watch to count the minutes), and check the time after every few questions to make sure you are "on schedule."

If you are forced to speed up, do it efficiently. Usually one or more answer choices can be eliminated without too much difficulty. Above all, don't panic. Don't speed up and just begin guessing at random choices. By pacing yourself, and continually monitoring your progress against your watch, you will always know exactly how far ahead or behind you are with your available time. If you find that you are one minute behind on the test, don't skip one question without spending any time on it, just to catch back up. Take 15 fewer seconds on the next four questions, and after four questions you'll have caught back up. Once you catch back up, you can continue working each problem at your normal pace.

Furthermore, don't dwell on the problems that you were rushed on. If a problem was taking up too much time and you made a hurried guess, it must be difficult. The difficult questions are the ones you are most likely to miss anyway, so it isn't a big loss. It is better to end with more time than you need than to run out of time.

Lastly, sometimes it is beneficial to slow down if you are constantly getting ahead of time. You are always more likely to catch a careless mistake by working more slowly than quickly, and among very high-scoring test takers (those who are likely to have lots of time left over), careless errors affect the score more than mastery of material.

Secret Key #2 - Guessing is not Guesswork

You probably know that guessing is a good idea. Unlike other standardized tests, there is no penalty for getting a wrong answer. Even if you have no idea about a question, you still have a 20-25% chance of getting it right.

Most test takers do not understand the impact that proper guessing can have on their score. Unless you score extremely high, guessing will significantly contribute to your final score.

Monkeys Take the Test

What most test takers don't realize is that to insure that 20-25% chance, you have to guess randomly. If you put 20 monkeys in a room to take this test, assuming they answered once per question and behaved themselves, on average they would get 20-25% of the questions correct. Put 20 test takers in the room, and the average will be much lower among guessed questions. Why?
1. The test writers intentionally write deceptive answer choices that "look" right. A test taker has no idea about a question, so he picks the "best looking" answer, which is often wrong. The monkey has no idea what looks good and what doesn't, so it will consistently be right about 20-25% of the time.
2. Test takers will eliminate answer choices from the guessing pool based on a hunch or intuition. Simple but correct answers often get excluded, leaving a 0% chance of being correct. The monkey has no clue, and often gets lucky with the best choice.

This is why the process of elimination endorsed by most test courses is flawed and detrimental to your performance. Test takers don't guess; they make an ignorant stab in the dark that is usually worse than random.

$5 Challenge

Let me introduce one of the most valuable ideas of this course—the $5 challenge:

You only mark your "best guess" if you are willing to bet $5 on it.
You only eliminate choices from guessing if you are willing to bet $5 on it.

Why $5? Five dollars is an amount of money that is small yet not insignificant, and can really add up fast (20 questions could cost you $100). Likewise, each answer choice on one question of the test will have a small impact on your overall score, but it can really add up to a lot of points in the end.

The process of elimination IS valuable. The following shows your chance of guessing it right:

If you eliminate wrong answer choices until only this many remain:	Chance of getting it correct:
1	100%
2	50%
3	33%

However, if you accidentally eliminate the right answer or go on a hunch for an incorrect answer, your chances drop dramatically—to 0%. By guessing among all the answer choices, you are GUARANTEED to have a shot at the right answer.

That's why the $5 test is so valuable. If you give up the advantage and safety of a pure guess, it had better be worth the risk.

What we still haven't covered is how to be sure that whatever guess you make is truly random. Here's the easiest way:

Always pick the first answer choice among those remaining.

Such a technique means that you have decided, **before you see a single test question**, exactly how you are going to guess, and since the order of choices tells you nothing about which one is correct, this guessing technique is perfectly random.

This section is not meant to scare you away from making educated guesses or eliminating choices; you just need to define when a choice is worth eliminating. The $5 test, along with a pre-defined random guessing strategy, is the best way to make sure you reap all of the benefits of guessing.

Secret Key #3 - Practice Smarter, Not Harder

Many test takers delay the test preparation process because they dread the awful amounts of practice time they think necessary to succeed on the test. We have refined an effective method that will take you only a fraction of the time.

There are a number of "obstacles" in the path to success. Among these are answering questions, finishing in time, and mastering test-taking strategies. All must be executed on the day of the test at peak performance, or your score will suffer. The test is a mental marathon that has a large impact on your future.

Just like a marathon runner, it is important to work your way up to the full challenge. So first you just worry about questions, and then time, and finally strategy:

Success Strategy

1. Find a good source for practice tests.
2. If you are willing to make a larger time investment, consider using more than one study guide. Often the different approaches of multiple authors will help you "get" difficult concepts.
3. Take a practice test with no time constraints, with all study helps, "open book." Take your time with questions and focus on applying strategies.
4. Take a practice test with time constraints, with all guides, "open book."
5. Take a final practice test without open material and with time limits.

If you have time to take more practice tests, just repeat step 5. By gradually exposing yourself to the full rigors of the test environment, you will condition your mind to the stress of test day and maximize your success.

Secret Key #4 - Prepare, Don't Procrastinate

Let me state an obvious fact: if you take the test three times, you will probably get three different scores. This is due to the way you feel on test day, the level of preparedness you have, and the version of the test you see. Despite the test writers' claims to the contrary, some versions of the test WILL be easier for you than others.

Since your future depends so much on your score, you should maximize your chances of success. In order to maximize the likelihood of success, you've got to prepare in advance. This means taking practice tests and spending time learning the information and test taking strategies you will need to succeed.

Never go take the actual test as a "practice" test, expecting that you can just take it again if you need to. Take all the practice tests you can on your own, but when you go to take the official test, be prepared, be focused, and do your best the first time!

Secret Key #5 - Test Yourself

Everyone knows that time is money. There is no need to spend too much of your time or too little of your time preparing for the test. You should only spend as much of your precious time preparing as is necessary for you to get the score you need.

Once you have taken a practice test under real conditions of time constraints, then you will know if you are ready for the test or not.

If you have scored extremely high the first time that you take the practice test, then there is not much point in spending countless hours studying. You are already there.

Benchmark your abilities by retaking practice tests and seeing how much you have improved. Once you consistently score high enough to guarantee success, then you are ready.

If you have scored well below where you need, then knuckle down and begin studying in earnest. Check your improvement regularly through the use of practice tests under real conditions. Above all, don't worry, panic, or give up. The key is perseverance!

Then, when you go to take the test, remain confident and remember how well you did on the practice tests. If you can score high enough on a practice test, then you can do the same on the real thing.

General Strategies

The most important thing you can do is to ignore your fears and jump into the test immediately. Do not be overwhelmed by any strange-sounding terms. You have to jump into the test like jumping into a pool—all at once is the easiest way.

Make Predictions

As you read and understand the question, try to guess what the answer will be. Remember that several of the answer choices are wrong, and once you begin reading them, your mind will immediately become cluttered with answer choices designed to throw you off. Your mind is typically the most focused immediately after you have read the question and digested its contents. If you can, try to predict what the correct answer will be. You may be surprised at what you can predict.

Quickly scan the choices and see if your prediction is in the listed answer choices. If it is, then you can be quite confident that you have the right answer. It still won't hurt to check the other answer choices, but most of the time, you've got it!

Answer the Question

It may seem obvious to only pick answer choices that answer the question, but the test writers can create some excellent answer choices that are wrong. Don't pick an answer just because it sounds right, or you believe it to be true. It MUST answer the question. Once you've made your selection, always go back and check it against the question and make sure that you didn't misread the question and that the answer choice does answer the question posed.

Benchmark

After you read the first answer choice, decide if you think it sounds correct or not. If it doesn't, move on to the next answer choice. If it does, mentally mark that answer choice. This doesn't mean that you've definitely selected it as your answer choice, it just means that it's the best you've seen thus far. Go ahead and read the next choice. If the next choice is worse than the one you've already selected, keep going to the next answer choice. If the next choice is better than the choice you've already selected, mentally mark the new answer choice as your best guess.

The first answer choice that you select becomes your standard. Every other answer choice must be benchmarked against that standard. That choice is correct until proven otherwise by another answer choice beating it out. Once you've decided that no other answer choice seems as good, do one final check to ensure that your answer choice answers the question posed.

Valid Information

Don't discount any of the information provided in the question. Every piece of information may be necessary to determine the correct answer. None of the information in the question is there to throw you off (while the answer choices will certainly have information to throw you off). If two seemingly unrelated topics are discussed, don't ignore either. You can be confident there is a relationship, or it wouldn't be included in the question, and you are probably going to have to determine what is that relationship to find the answer.

Avoid "Fact Traps"

Don't get distracted by a choice that is factually true. Your search is for the answer that answers the question. Stay focused and don't fall for an answer that is true but irrelevant. Always go back to the question and make sure you're choosing an answer that actually answers the question and is not just a true statement. An answer can be factually correct, but it MUST answer the question asked. Additionally, two answers can both be seemingly correct, so be sure to read all of the answer choices, and make sure that you get the one that BEST answers the question.

Milk the Question

Some of the questions may throw you completely off. They might deal with a subject you have not been exposed to, or one that you haven't reviewed in years. While your lack of knowledge about the subject will be a hindrance, the question itself can give you many clues that will help you find the correct answer. Read the question carefully and look for clues. Watch particularly for adjectives and nouns describing difficult terms or words that you don't recognize. Regardless of whether you completely understand a word or not, replacing it with a synonym, either provided or one you more familiar with, may help you to understand what the questions are asking. Rather than wracking your mind about specific detailed information concerning a difficult term or word, try to use mental substitutes that are easier to understand.

The Trap of Familiarity

Don't just choose a word because you recognize it. On difficult questions, you may not recognize a number of words in the answer choices. The test writers don't put "make-believe" words on the test, so don't think that just because you only recognize all the words in one answer choice that that answer choice must be correct. If you only recognize words in one answer choice, then focus on that one. Is it correct? Try your best to determine if it is correct. If it is, that's great. If not, eliminate it. Each word and answer choice you eliminate increases your chances of getting the question correct, even if you then have to guess among the unfamiliar choices.

Eliminate Answers

Eliminate choices as soon as you realize they are wrong. But be careful! Make sure you consider all of the possible answer choices. Just because one appears right, doesn't mean that the next one won't be even better! The test writers will usually put more than one good answer choice for every question, so read all of them. Don't worry if you are stuck between two that seem right. By getting down to just two remaining possible choices, your odds are now 50/50. Rather than wasting too much time, play the odds. You are guessing, but guessing wisely because you've been able to knock out some of the answer choices that you know are wrong. If you are eliminating choices and realize that the last answer choice you are left with is also obviously wrong, don't panic. Start over and consider each choice again. There may easily be something that you missed the first time and will realize on the second pass.

Tough Questions

If you are stumped on a problem or it appears too hard or too difficult, don't waste time. Move on! Remember though, if you can quickly check for obviously incorrect answer choices, your chances of guessing correctly are greatly improved. Before you completely give up, at least try to knock out a couple of possible answers. Eliminate what you can and then guess at the remaining answer choices before moving on.

Brainstorm

If you get stuck on a difficult question, spend a few seconds quickly brainstorming. Run through the complete list of possible answer choices. Look at each choice and ask yourself, "Could this answer the question satisfactorily?" Go through each answer choice and consider it independently of the others. By systematically going through all possibilities, you may find something that you would otherwise overlook. Remember though that when you get stuck, it's important to try to keep moving.

Read Carefully

Understand the problem. Read the question and answer choices carefully. Don't miss the question because you misread the terms. You have plenty of time to read each question thoroughly and make sure you understand what is being asked. Yet a happy medium must be attained, so don't waste too much time. You must read carefully, but efficiently.

Face Value

When in doubt, use common sense. Always accept the situation in the problem at face value. Don't read too much into it. These problems will not require you to make huge leaps of logic. The test writers aren't trying to throw you off with a cheap trick. If you have to go beyond creativity and make a leap of logic in order to have an answer choice answer the question, then you should look at the other answer choices. Don't overcomplicate the problem by creating theoretical relationships or explanations that will warp time or space. These are normal problems rooted in reality. It's just that the applicable relationship or explanation may not be readily apparent and you have to figure things out. Use your common sense to interpret anything that isn't clear.

Prefixes

If you're having trouble with a word in the question or answer choices, try dissecting it. Take advantage of every clue that the word might include. Prefixes and suffixes can be a huge help. Usually they allow you to determine a basic meaning. Pre- means before, post- means after, pro - is positive, de- is negative. From these prefixes and suffixes, you can get an idea of the general meaning of the word and try to put it into context. Beware though of any traps. Just because con- is the opposite of pro-, doesn't necessarily mean congress is the opposite of progress!

Hedge Phrases

Watch out for critical hedge phrases, led off with words such as "likely," "may," "can," "sometimes," "often," "almost," "mostly," "usually," "generally," "rarely," and "sometimes." Question writers insert these hedge phrases to cover every possibility. Often an answer choice will be wrong simply because it leaves no room for exception. Unless the situation calls for them, avoid answer choices that have definitive words like "exactly," and "always."

Switchback Words

Stay alert for "switchbacks." These are the words and phrases frequently used to alert you to shifts in thought. The most common switchback word is "but." Others include "although," "however," "nevertheless," "on the other hand," "even though," "while," "in spite of," "despite," and "regardless of."

New Information

Correct answer choices will rarely have completely new information included. Answer choices typically are straightforward reflections of the material asked about and will directly relate to the question. If a new piece of information is included in an answer choice that doesn't even seem to relate to the topic being asked about, then that answer choice is likely incorrect. All of the information needed to answer the question is usually provided for you in the question. You should not have to make guesses that are unsupported or choose answer choices that require unknown information that cannot be reasoned from what is given.

Time Management

On technical questions, don't get lost on the technical terms. Don't spend too much time on any one question. If you don't know what a term means, then odds are you aren't going to get much further since you don't have a dictionary. You should be able to immediately recognize whether or not you know a term. If you don't, work with the other clues that you have—the other answer choices and terms provided—but don't waste too much time trying to figure out a difficult term that you don't know.

Contextual Clues

Look for contextual clues. An answer can be right but not the correct answer. The contextual clues will help you find the answer that is most right and is correct. Understand the context in which a phrase or statement is made. This will help you make important distinctions.

Don't Panic

Panicking will not answer any questions for you; therefore, it isn't helpful. When you first see the question, if your mind goes blank, take a deep breath. Force yourself to mechanically go through the steps of solving the problem using the strategies you've learned.

Pace Yourself

Don't get clock fever. It's easy to be overwhelmed when you're looking at a page full of questions, your mind is full of random thoughts and feeling confused, and the clock is ticking down faster than you would like. Calm down and maintain the pace that you have set for yourself. As long as you are on track by monitoring your pace, you are guaranteed to have enough time for yourself. When you get to the last few minutes of the test, it may seem like you won't have enough time left, but if you only have as many questions as you should have left at that point, then you're right on track!

Answer Selection

The best way to pick an answer choice is to eliminate all of those that are wrong, until only one is left and confirm that is the correct answer. Sometimes though, an answer choice may immediately look right. Be careful! Take a second to make sure that the other choices are not equally obvious. Don't make a hasty mistake. There are only two times that you should stop before checking other answers. First is when you are positive that the answer choice you have selected is correct. Second is when time is almost out and you have to make a quick guess!

Check Your Work

Since you will probably not know every term listed and the answer to every question, it is important that you get credit for the ones that you do know. Don't miss any questions through careless mistakes. If at all possible, try to take a second to look back over your answer selection and make sure you've selected the correct answer choice and haven't made a costly careless mistake (such as marking an answer choice that you didn't mean to mark). The time it takes for this quick double check should more than pay for itself in caught mistakes.

Beware of Directly Quoted Answers

Sometimes an answer choice will repeat word for word a portion of the question or reference section. However, beware of such exact duplication. It may be a trap! More than likely, the correct choice will paraphrase or summarize a point, rather than being exactly the same wording.

Slang

Scientific sounding answers are better than slang ones. An answer choice that begins "To compare the outcomes..." is much more likely to be correct than one that begins "Because some people insisted..."

Extreme Statements

Avoid wild answers that throw out highly controversial ideas that are proclaimed as established fact. An answer choice that states the "process should used in certain situations, if..." is much more likely to be correct than one that states the "process should be discontinued completely." The first is a calm rational statement and doesn't even make a definitive, uncompromising stance, using a hedge word "if" to provide wiggle room, whereas the second choice is a radical idea and far more extreme.

Answer Choice Families

When you have two or more answer choices that are direct opposites or parallels, one of them is usually the correct answer. For instance, if one answer choice states "x increases" and another answer choice states "x decreases" or "y increases," then those two or three answer choices are very similar in construction and fall into the same family of answer choices. A family of answer choices consists of two or three answer choices, very similar in construction, but often with directly opposite meanings. Usually the correct answer choice will be in that family of answer choices. The "odd man out" or answer choice that doesn't seem to fit the parallel construction of the other answer choices is more likely to be incorrect.

Special Report: How to Overcome Test Anxiety

The very nature of tests caters to some level of anxiety, nervousness, or tension, just as we feel for any important event that occurs in our lives. A little bit of anxiety or nervousness can be a good thing. It helps us with motivation, and makes achievement just that much sweeter. However, too much anxiety can be a problem, especially if it hinders our ability to function and perform.

"Test anxiety," is the term that refers to the emotional reactions that some test-takers experience when faced with a test or exam. Having a fear of testing and exams is based upon a rational fear, since the test-taker's performance can shape the course of an academic career. Nevertheless, experiencing excessive fear of examinations will only interfere with the test-taker's ability to perform and chance to be successful.

There are a large variety of causes that can contribute to the development and sensation of test anxiety. These include, but are not limited to, lack of preparation and worrying about issues surrounding the test.

Lack of Preparation

Lack of preparation can be identified by the following behaviors or situations:

- Not scheduling enough time to study, and therefore cramming the night before the test or exam
- Managing time poorly, to create the sensation that there is not enough time to do everything
- Failing to organize the text information in advance, so that the study material consists of the entire text and not simply the pertinent information
- Poor overall studying habits

Worrying, on the other hand, can be related to both the test taker, or many other factors around him/her that will be affected by the results of the test. These include worrying about:

- Previous performances on similar exams, or exams in general
- How friends and other students are achieving
- The negative consequences that will result from a poor grade or failure

There are three primary elements to test anxiety. Physical components, which involve the same typical bodily reactions as those to acute anxiety (to be discussed below). Emotional factors have to do with fear or panic. Mental or cognitive issues concerning attention spans and memory abilities.

Physical Signals

There are many different symptoms of test anxiety, and these are not limited to mental and emotional strain. Frequently there are a range of physical signals that will let a test taker know that he/she is suffering from test anxiety. These bodily changes can include the following:

- Perspiring
- Sweaty palms
- Wet, trembling hands
- Nausea
- Dry mouth
- A knot in the stomach
- Headache
- Faintness
- Muscle tension
- Aching shoulders, back and neck
- Rapid heart beat
- Feeling too hot/cold

To recognize the sensation of test anxiety, a test-taker should monitor him/herself for the following sensations:

- The physical distress symptoms as listed above
- Emotional sensitivity, expressing emotional feelings such as the need to cry or laugh too much, or a sensation of anger or helplessness
- A decreased ability to think, causing the test-taker to blank out or have racing thoughts that are hard to organize or control.

Though most students will feel some level of anxiety when faced with a test or exam, the majority can cope with that anxiety and maintain it at a manageable level. However, those who cannot are faced with a very real and very serious condition, which can and should be controlled for the immeasurable benefit of this sufferer.

Naturally, these sensations lead to negative results for the testing experience. The most common effects of test anxiety have to do with nervousness and mental blocking.

Nervousness

Nervousness can appear in several different levels:

- The test-taker's difficulty, or even inability to read and understand the questions on the test
- The difficulty or inability to organize thoughts to a coherent form
- The difficulty or inability to recall key words and concepts relating to the testing questions (especially essays)
- The receipt of poor grades on a test, though the test material was well known by the test taker

Conversely, a person may also experience mental blocking, which involves:

- Blanking out on test questions
- Only remembering the correct answers to the questions when the test has already finished.

Fortunately for test anxiety sufferers, beating these feelings, to a large degree, has to do with proper preparation. When a test taker has a feeling of preparedness, then anxiety will be dramatically lessened.

The first step to resolving anxiety issues is to distinguish which of the two types of anxiety are being suffered. If the anxiety is a direct result of a lack of preparation, this should be considered a normal reaction, and the anxiety level (as opposed to the test results) shouldn't be anything to worry about. However, if, when adequately prepared, the test-taker still panics, blanks out, or seems to overreact, this is not a fully rational reaction. While this can be considered normal too, there are many ways to combat and overcome these effects.

Remember that anxiety cannot be entirely eliminated, however, there are ways to minimize it, to make the anxiety easier to manage. Preparation is one of the best ways to minimize test anxiety. Therefore the following techniques are wise in order to best fight off any anxiety that may want to build.

To begin with, try to avoid cramming before a test, whenever it is possible. By trying to memorize an entire term's worth of information in one day, you'll be shocking your system, and not giving yourself a very good chance to absorb the information. This is an easy path to anxiety, so for those who suffer from test anxiety, cramming should not even be considered an option.

Instead of cramming, work throughout the semester to combine all of the material which is presented throughout the semester, and work on it gradually as the course goes by, making sure to master the main concepts first, leaving minor details for a week or so before the test.

To study for the upcoming exam, be sure to pose questions that may be on the examination, to gauge the ability to answer them by integrating the ideas from your texts, notes and lectures, as well as any supplementary readings.

If it is truly impossible to cover all of the information that was covered in that particular term, concentrate on the most important portions, that can be covered very well. Learn these concepts as best as possible, so that when the test comes, a goal can be made to use these concepts as presentations of your knowledge.

In addition to study habits, changes in attitude are critical to beating a struggle with test anxiety. In fact, an improvement of the perspective over the entire test-taking experience can actually help a test taker to enjoy studying and therefore improve the overall experience. Be certain not to overemphasize the significance of the grade - know that the result of the test is neither a reflection of self worth, nor is it a measure of intelligence; one grade will not predict a person's future success.

To improve an overall testing outlook, the following steps should be tried:

- Keeping in mind that the most reasonable expectation for taking a test is to expect to try to demonstrate as much of what you know as you possibly can.
- Reminding ourselves that a test is only one test; this is not the only one, and there will be others.
- The thought of thinking of oneself in an irrational, all-or-nothing term should be avoided at all costs.
- A reward should be designated for after the test, so there's something to look forward to. Whether it be going to a movie, going out to eat, or simply visiting friends, schedule it in advance, and do it no matter what result is expected on the exam.

Test-takers should also keep in mind that the basics are some of the most important things, even beyond anti-anxiety techniques and studying. Never neglect the basic social, emotional and biological needs, in order to try to absorb information. In order to best achieve, these three factors must be held as just as important as the studying itself.

Study Steps

Remember the following important steps for studying:

- Maintain healthy nutrition and exercise habits. Continue both your recreational activities and social pass times. These both contribute to your physical and emotional well being.
- Be certain to get a good amount of sleep, especially the night before the test, because when you're overtired you are not able to perform to the best of your best ability.
- Keep the studying pace to a moderate level by taking breaks when they are needed, and varying the work whenever possible, to keep the mind fresh instead of getting bored.
- When enough studying has been done that all the material that can be learned has been learned, and the test taker is prepared for the test, stop studying and do something relaxing such as listening to music, watching a movie, or taking a warm bubble bath.

There are also many other techniques to minimize the uneasiness or apprehension that is experienced along with test anxiety before, during, or even after the examination. In fact, there are a great deal of things that can be done to stop anxiety from interfering with lifestyle and performance. Again, remember that anxiety will not be eliminated entirely, and it shouldn't be. Otherwise that "up" feeling for exams would not exist, and most of us depend on that sensation to perform better than usual. However, this anxiety has to be at a level that is manageable.

Of course, as we have just discussed, being prepared for the exam is half the battle right away. Attending all classes, finding out what knowledge will be expected on the exam, and knowing the exam schedules are easy steps to lowering anxiety. Keeping up with work will remove the need to cram, and efficient study habits will eliminate wasted time. Studying should be done in an ideal location for concentration, so that it is simple to become interested in the material and give it complete attention. A method such as SQ3R (Survey, Question, Read, Recite, Review) is a wonderful key to follow to make sure that the study habits are as effective as possible, especially in the case of learning from a textbook. Flashcards are great techniques for memorization. Learning to take good notes will mean that notes will be full of useful information, so that less sifting will need to be done to seek out what is pertinent for studying. Reviewing notes after class and then again on occasion will keep the information fresh in the mind. From notes that have been taken summary sheets and outlines can be made for simpler reviewing.

A study group can also be a very motivational and helpful place to study, as there will be a sharing of ideas, all of the minds can work together, to make sure that everyone understands, and the studying will be made more interesting because it will be a social occasion.

Basically, though, as long as the test-taker remains organized and self confident, with efficient study habits, less time will need to be spent studying, and higher grades will be achieved.

To become self confident, there are many useful steps. The first of these is "self talk." It has been shown through extensive research, that self-talk for students who suffer from test anxiety, should be well monitored, in order to make sure that it contributes to self confidence as opposed to sinking the student. Frequently the self talk of test-anxious students is negative or self-defeating, thinking that everyone else is smarter and faster, that they always mess up, and that if they don't do well, they'll fail the entire course. It is important to decreasing anxiety that awareness is made of self talk. Try writing any negative self thoughts and then disputing them with a positive statement instead. Begin self-encouragement as though it was a friend speaking. Repeat positive statements to help reprogram the mind to believing in successes instead of failures.

Helpful Techniques

Other extremely helpful techniques include:

- Self-visualization of doing well and reaching goals
- While aiming for an "A" level of understanding, don't try to "overprotect" by setting your expectations lower. This will only convince the mind to stop studying in order to meet the lower expectations.
- Don't make comparisons with the results or habits of other students. These are individual factors, and different things work for different people, causing different results.
- Strive to become an expert in learning what works well, and what can be done in order to improve. Consider collecting this data in a journal.
- Create rewards for after studying instead of doing things before studying that will only turn into avoidance behaviors.
- Make a practice of relaxing - by using methods such as progressive relaxation, self-hypnosis, guided imagery, etc - in order to make relaxation an automatic sensation.
- Work on creating a state of relaxed concentration so that concentrating will take on the focus of the mind, so that none will be wasted on worrying.
- Take good care of the physical self by eating well and getting enough sleep.
- Plan in time for exercise and stick to this plan.

Beyond these techniques, there are other methods to be used before, during and after the test that will help the test-taker perform well in addition to overcoming anxiety.

Before the exam comes the academic preparation. This involves establishing a study schedule and beginning at least one week before the actual date of the test. By doing this, the anxiety of not having enough time to study for the test will be automatically eliminated. Moreover, this will make the studying a much more effective experience, ensuring that the learning will be an easier process. This relieves much undue pressure on the test-taker.

Summary sheets, note cards, and flash cards with the main concepts and examples of these main concepts should be prepared in advance of the actual studying time. A topic should never be eliminated from this process. By omitting a topic because it isn't expected to be on the test is only setting up the test-taker for anxiety should it actually appear on the exam. Utilize the course syllabus for laying out the topics that should be studied. Carefully go over the notes that were made in class, paying special attention to any of the issues that the professor took special care to emphasize while lecturing in class. In the textbooks, use the chapter review, or if possible, the chapter tests, to begin your review.

It may even be possible to ask the instructor what information will be covered on the exam, or what the format of the exam will be (for example, multiple choice, essay, free form, true-false). Additionally, see if it is possible to find out how many questions will be on the test. If a review sheet or sample test has been offered by the professor, make good use of it, above anything else, for the preparation for the test. Another great resource for getting to know the examination is reviewing tests from previous semesters. Use these tests to review, and aim to achieve a 100% score on each of the possible topics. With a few exceptions, the goal that you set for yourself is the highest one that you will reach.

Take all of the questions that were assigned as homework, and rework them to any other possible course material. The more problems reworked, the more skill and confidence will form as a result. When forming the solution to a problem, write out each of the steps. Don't simply do head work. By doing as many steps on paper as possible, much clarification and therefore confidence will be formed. Do this with as many homework problems as possible, before checking the answers. By checking the answer after each problem, a reinforcement will exist, that will not be on the exam. Study situations should be as exam-like as possible, to prime the test-taker's system for the experience. By waiting to check the answers at the end, a psychological advantage will be formed, to decrease the stress factor.

Another fantastic reason for not cramming is the avoidance of confusion in concepts, especially when it comes to mathematics. 8-10 hours of study will become one hundred percent more effective if it is spread out over a week or at least several days, instead of doing it all in one sitting. Recognize that the human brain requires time in order to assimilate new material, so frequent breaks and a span of study time over several days will be much more beneficial.

Additionally, don't study right up until the point of the exam. Studying should stop a minimum of one hour before the exam begins. This allows the brain to rest and put things in their proper order. This will also provide the time to become as relaxed as possible when going into the examination room. The test-taker will also have time to eat well and eat sensibly. Know that the brain needs food as much as the rest of the body. With enough food and enough sleep, as well as a relaxed attitude, the body and the mind are primed for success.

Avoid any anxious classmates who are talking about the exam. These students only spread anxiety, and are not worth sharing the anxious sentimentalities.

Before the test also involves creating a positive attitude, so mental preparation should also be a point of concentration. There are many keys to creating a positive attitude. Should fears become rushing in, make a visualization of taking the exam, doing well, and seeing an A written on the paper. Write out a list of affirmations that will bring a feeling of confidence, such as "I am doing well in my English class," "I studied well and know my material," "I enjoy this class." Even if the affirmations aren't believed at first, it sends a positive message to the subconscious which will result in an alteration of the overall belief system, which is the system that creates reality.

If a sensation of panic begins, work with the fear and imagine the very worst! Work through the entire scenario of not passing the test, failing the entire course, and dropping out of school, followed by not getting a job, and pushing a shopping cart through the dark alley where you'll live. This will place things into perspective! Then, practice deep breathing and create a visualization of the opposite situation - achieving an "A" on the exam, passing the entire course, receiving the degree at a graduation ceremony.

On the day of the test, there are many things to be done to ensure the best results, as well as the most calm outlook. The following stages are suggested in order to maximize test-taking potential:

- Begin the examination day with a moderate breakfast, and avoid any coffee or beverages with caffeine if the test taker is prone to jitters. Even people who are used to managing caffeine can feel jittery or light-headed when it is taken on a test day.
- Attempt to do something that is relaxing before the examination begins. As last minute cramming clouds the mastering of overall concepts, it is better to use this time to create a calming outlook.
- Be certain to arrive at the test location well in advance, in order to provide time to select a location that is away from doors, windows and other distractions, as well as giving enough time to relax before the test begins.
- Keep away from anxiety generating classmates who will upset the sensation of stability and relaxation that is being attempted before the exam.
- Should the waiting period before the exam begins cause anxiety, create a self-distraction by reading a light magazine or something else that is relaxing and simple.

During the exam itself, read the entire exam from beginning to end, and find out how much time should be allotted to each individual problem. Once writing the exam, should more time be taken for a problem, it should be abandoned, in order to begin another problem. If there is time at the end, the unfinished problem can always be returned to and completed.

Read the instructions very carefully - twice - so that unpleasant surprises won't follow during or after the exam has ended.

When writing the exam, pretend that the situation is actually simply the completion of homework within a library, or at home. This will assist in forming a relaxed atmosphere, and will allow the brain extra focus for the complex thinking function.

Begin the exam with all of the questions with which the most confidence is felt. This will build the confidence level regarding the entire exam and will begin a quality momentum. This will also create encouragement for trying the problems where uncertainty resides.

Going with the "gut instinct" is always the way to go when solving a problem. Second guessing should be avoided at all costs. Have confidence in the ability to do well.

For essay questions, create an outline in advance that will keep the mind organized and make certain that all of the points are remembered. For multiple choice, read every answer, even if the correct one has been spotted - a better one may exist.

Continue at a pace that is reasonable and not rushed, in order to be able to work carefully. Provide enough time to go over the answers at the end, to check for small errors that can be corrected.

Should a feeling of panic begin, breathe deeply, and think of the feeling of the body releasing sand through its pores. Visualize a calm, peaceful place, and include all of the sights, sounds and sensations of this image. Continue the deep breathing, and take a few minutes to continue this with closed eyes. When all is well again, return to the test.

If a "blanking" occurs for a certain question, skip it and move on to the next question. There will be time to return to the other question later. Get everything done that can be done, first, to guarantee all the grades that can be compiled, and to build all of the confidence possible. Then return to the weaker questions to build the marks from there.

Remember, one's own reality can be created, so as long as the belief is there, success will follow. And remember: anxiety can happen later, right now, there's an exam to be written!

After the examination is complete, whether there is a feeling for a good grade or a bad grade, don't dwell on the exam, and be certain to follow through on the reward that was promised...and enjoy it! Don't dwell on any mistakes that have been made, as there is nothing that can be done at this point anyway.

Additionally, don't begin to study for the next test right away. Do something relaxing for a while, and let the mind relax and prepare itself to begin absorbing information again.

From the results of the exam - both the grade and the entire experience, be certain to learn from what has gone on. Perfect studying habits and work some more on confidence in order to make the next examination experience even better than the last one.

Learn to avoid places where openings occurred for laziness, procrastination and day dreaming.

Use the time between this exam and the next one to better learn to relax, even learning to relax on cue, so that any anxiety can be controlled during the next exam. Learn how to relax the body. Slouch in your chair if that helps. Tighten and then relax all of the different muscle groups, one group at a time, beginning with the feet and then working all the way up to the neck and face. This will ultimately relax the muscles more than they were to begin with. Learn how to breathe deeply and comfortably, and focus on this breathing going in and out as a relaxing thought. With every exhale, repeat the word "relax."

As common as test anxiety is, it is very possible to overcome it. Make yourself one of the test-takers who overcome this frustrating hindrance.

Additional Bonus Material

Due to our efforts to try to keep this book to a manageable length, we've created a link that will give you access to all of your additional bonus material.

Please visit http://www.mometrix.com/bonus948/certdiabedu to access the information.